Palliative Care for (

)a
Royal Cornwall Hospital
Treliske
Truro. TR1 3HD

Palliative Care for Care Homes

A PRACTICAL HANDBOOK

CHRISTINE REDDALL

Macmillan Nurse for Care Homes
NHS Warwickshire

Foreword by

PROFESSOR TIM HUNT MD, PhD, FRCP
Emeritus Consultant in Palliative Medicine
Brookfields Hospital, Cambridge
EU Professor in Special Medicine

Radcliffe Publishing
Oxford • New York

Radcliffe Publishing Ltd
18 Marcham Road
Abingdon
Oxon OX14 1AA
United Kingdom

www.radcliffe-oxford.com
Electronic catalogue and worldwide online ordering facility.

British Library Cataloguing in Publication Data

A catalogue record for this book is available from the British Library.

ISBN-13: 978 184619 248 7

Typeset by Pindar NZ, Auckland, New Zealand
Printed and bound by TJI Digital, Padstow, Cornwall, UK

Contents

Foreword

The growing and undisputed importance of care homes in today's social fabric cannot be exaggerated. This book is directed at carers who are at the front-line of such care. Here we have a text for those who want to roll up their sleeves to look after those in care homes. It is not for the theoretician and avoids the vacillation and pontifical writing often associated with palliative care. A strong practical approach is stamped throughout the book in a language and style to embrace carers. It is written by someone who has immersed herself in actual empathetic practical care. Her extraordinary keenness and warmth radiate from each page, and her very personal approach, while alien to much professional expression, is written without discomfiture as she writes about her father, his illness and death. It is these penetrating personal experiences that fuel her motivation to understand and help other carers.

Many avert their eyes from the silent suffering and often distressing situations that we may witness in care homes and many forget the praise and respect which we should accord to carers. We owe much to others, especially to the older person. They have nurtured us and striven to give us a better life than they experienced; they have fought for our relative freedom and each of us tomorrow will need care.

This book will help the elderly, all persons in our care, their relatives and close friends and above all the carers who deserve our unstinted support and unreserved acclamation.

Professor Tim Hunt MD, PhD, FRCP
Emeritus Consultant in Palliative Medicine
Brookfields Hospital, Cambridge
EU Professor in Special Medicine
October 2008

Preface

This is a resource book that provides information on palliative care. It is designed primarily to help carers who work in care homes of all categories. To my knowledge, it is the first book written solely for carers working in care homes that addresses the issues of caring for individuals with palliative care needs. However, people to whom I have spoken about this book, or who have read parts of it, have all said that it would also be a helpful resource for non-professional family carers who are caring for a family member in their own home.

The book is designed to be readable by all levels of carers, and I have endeavoured to keep the language and text as 'non-medical' as possible. I have pondered over the most appropriate name for the groups of people I shall be discussing in this book, as it is necessary to maintain consistency of that name throughout the text. In the various care homes that I visit in my work, 'patients' are referred to as 'residents', 'clients' and 'service users'. 'Carers' are variously referred to as sisters, matrons, staff nurses, auxiliary nurses and support workers. Therefore, for ease of reading, I have chosen to refer to all those who care for people as 'carers', and all those who receive care as 'patients.' When referring to an individual, I use either gender indiscriminately. All illnesses that fall within the category of palliative care are referred to as 'life limiting.'

In this book, each chapter explores an aspect of palliative care in relation to the type of patients who are cared for in a care home, and the carers who provide this care on a daily basis. The reader can of course dip in and out of the various chapters according to the information that they need at the time.

My background is in nursing, and at the time of writing I have been a nurse for 37 years. I started off as most nurses do, working on a variety of wards, gaining experience and deciding which areas of nursing I found most rewarding. I soon settled into care of the elderly – known as 'geriatrics' in those days. Through working in this area, I developed an interest in palliative care and embarked on a career path that would eventually gain me a post as a Macmillan nurse. The path was not easy, and involved doing courses, obtaining a degree, writing articles, getting myself known and applying for jobs. My determination eventually paid off, and in 1995 I obtained my first post as a Macmillan nurse. Since then, my passion for palliative care has gone from strength to strength, and at the time of writing I am employed by Warwickshire NHS Trust, working as a Macmillan nurse for care homes across Warwickshire. I have a combined clinical and educational remit, and find myself in a thoroughly rewarding job that combines my two favourite areas of nursing – palliative care and care of the elderly. It is this role that has prompted me to write this book. While meeting the many carers who work in the homes, and providing them with palliative care education, I have listened closely to their needs. It is my belief that the skills possessed by these carers who work in care homes, and the care that they provide for our ever increasing elderly population, are often underestimated. (I should add here that although the elderly make up the largest proportion of residents in care homes, increasing numbers of younger people are being cared for in these establishments. Indeed, of the 21 care home residents currently on my caseload, three are under 50 years of age.)

During my early nursing years I worked mainly with the elderly, and although I found this both interesting and rewarding, compared with my colleagues who were working in Accident and Emergency and other more acute settings, I was often made to feel that I was working in a 'backwater' area of nursing. 'Geriatric nursing' was seen as easy, not requiring much in the way of brain power, and a thankless task.

However, over the years, I have come to realise that the elderly in particular often have very complex needs, as they are generally suffering from more than one illness, and frequently taking a cocktail of medication that has been added to over the years. It also became apparent to me that caring for elderly people during their illness requires very special skills, such as the need to be aware of a host of different diseases, different medications and dose ranges, and the need to deal with mental and physical impairment.

Because of the ageing general population, more and more care homes are finding themselves caring for patients with complex life-limiting conditions, such as cancer, motor neurone disease, diabetes, stroke and heart failure, to name just a few. This is happening even in the care homes (sometimes called 'residential homes') where the carers are mostly untrained. There are also many homes where carers help to support people with learning disabilities.

These types of home are often conventional houses situated in residential areas, usually housing an average of between two to eight residents with learning disabilities plus live in carer(s).

Care homes must observe many rules and regulations which are laid down by their governing body. Much of their training (e.g. in lifting and handling, wound care and food hygiene) is mandatory. However, despite the increasing numbers of patients in care homes who are suffering from a range of life-limiting illnesses (such as those mentioned above), palliative care training is not mandatory. It has therefore been very enlightening to find that, since working within this role, I have been inundated with requests to provide palliative care training. I have been astounded by the amount of interest in palliative care, to the extent that many nurses attend unpaid education sessions, in their own time, and often after working a night shift. While providing these education sessions, it became apparent to me that carers are often unclear about the real meaning of 'palliative care', many believing that palliative care refers specifically to care given to a person who has cancer, or during the final days of life. Confusion also surrounds the role of the Macmillan nurse and the hospice, and how the various services that come under the umbrella of palliative care work together. The more I have visited and helped to support care homes in my capacity as a Macmillan nurse, the more I have discovered about the care that is provided in these environments, and how isolated many of the carers are from study days, sources of new information and other resources to keep them up to date.

I am aware that for huge numbers of care homes around the UK there may seldom be the opportunity to undertake training in palliative care, and although the situation is a lot better than it used to be, there are still not many nurses currently working in roles similar to mine. Hence the need for this book!

The content of this book is not new. It is not full of mind-blowing technology or medical jargon, it does not contain a great deal of referenced material, nor does it include many charts or facts and figures. Much of the information in this book can be sourced elsewhere. You could buy a palliative care book on symptom control, communication, cancer, etc. You could send away for literature about Macmillan nurses, hospices and benefits. Or, if you are computer literate, you could find all kinds of information about palliative care on the Internet. What I have done is to pool all the information together in one book, using information drawn on my own experience of palliative care in this area, backed up by case histories of real people (their names have been changed, of course) and my experience of working closely with a large number of carers. I have tried to put myself in the shoes of carers, especially those without medical training, and to consider what they might want to know when caring for patients with a life-limiting illness.

I know that care homes often receive much criticism from various sources, and, as in every walk of life, there is good and not so good practice. However, I have to say that during my current role, I have seen far more good than bad. Since I have been working in this area, it has been a real privilege to help to convey the principles and practice of palliative care to the carers who work in care homes. The provision of good general palliative care that has prevented a patient from being admitted to hospital in their last days of life is a huge achievement that should always be applauded.

So, to all carers who are dedicated to working in a care home, I take my hat off to you. If you are one of these carers, just by getting hold of this book you are showing interest and compassion in your caring role. So take heart – you do a great job and provide care for a wide range of patients with differing needs. Read the book, boost your confidence and carry on doing a good job.

Christine Reddall
October 2008

About the author

Christine has been a qualified nurse since 1973. Having spent a large part of her nursing career in care of the elderly, she developed a passion for palliative care and her ultimate goal was to become a Macmillan nurse. She achieved this goal in 1997, following completion of a degree in palliative care. After working as a community Macmillan nurse for 7 years, she was delighted to be appointed Macmillan Nurse for Care Homes across Warwickshire. This was a brand new post, with a 50% clinical and 50% educational remit. Over the past 4 years, Christine has focused on developing this service and enhancing the palliative care that is delivered in care homes. Some of her work has been published in nursing journals, but this is her first book.

Acknowledgements

I would like to thank all of the care homes across Warwickshire that have given me such a wonderful insight into the care that they provide for their patients. You know who you are, and I think you are wonderful.

I wish to thank my sister Sue and friends Carol and Barbara for proofreading each chapter as I went along. As non-medical people, their input was valuable in helping to prevent this book from becoming too medical. If they didn't understand something, it wasn't included!

A special thank you is due to my daughter Lisa, for formatting the manuscript.

I also owe a big thank you to my husband Phil, for his encouragement and constant nagging to 'turn off my work phone' so that I could get down to writing. He also painstakingly reproduced my hand-drawn charts in formats that could be printed.

I would like to remember a very special friend, Frankie, who died in a care home in 2006 aged 99 years. She was suffering from a life-limiting illness, yet she bore it with dignity and a smile (most of the time). Despite her frailty, she was a strong voice when it came to deciding how she wanted to be cared for, and I know she will be long remembered by all who had the privilege of caring for her.

Dedication

This book is dedicated to my father, who died from mesothelioma in March 2006. I know that if he were alive today he would be so proud that I had written this book.

His illness is part of the reason why I chose to write in the way that I have. Like myself, Dad's family and friends struggled to understand what was happening to him, and what they could do to help. My mother was with him when he died, and she has struggled to come to terms with what happened at the end. Of course I struggled, too, but in a different way. Like my family, I hated seeing what the illness was doing to my father, and I hated the fact that he was going to die, but unlike my family, I struggled because I knew so much about his illness and I knew what was happening. In some ways, having this knowledge both hindered and helped me. It hindered me because I just wanted to be a daughter – not a nurse. However, it also helped me because I knew what the disease was doing to him, and I was able to help my family to understand this as well.

Because this book is dedicated to my father, I would like to tell you about our wonderful trip together.

Dad's two loves in life were his family and going on holiday. He and my mother had recently celebrated their diamond wedding anniversary and were enjoying a holiday with myself and my husband on a short visit to Amsterdam. We were talking about holidays when my father voiced a wish to go to India to see a tiger. After much joking about the easier option of going to London Zoo, my well-travelled, active, 82-year-old mother decided that this type of jungle adventure was a little beyond her capabilities. So I, having the same sense of adventure as my father, and at the tender age of 53 years, said that I would love to go with him. As soon as we arrived home from Amsterdam, my father embarked on a trawl of holiday brochures and trips to the library to research the area. He finally decided on a trip to Nepal that included a search for the Bengal tiger! He took great pleasure in organising everything for us, and as I was still working, I willingly left him to it. We eventually received our date of departure – 21 February 2005. We flew business class and enjoyed the luxury of this, as it was a new experience for both of us. In Kathmandu, we met up with our fellow travellers and our guide. My father and I went on elephant safaris at the crack of dawn, flew over Mount Everest, went horse riding (my father's first and only experience of this), and saw the magnificent sight of the sun rising over the Annapurna mountain range. While we were waiting to get on a river boat, a rhinoceros appeared out of the bushes. Our guide told us not to panic, but said that if it did charge, we must all run in the opposite direction, throwing off items of clothing to distract it! Fortunately, it didn't charge and we all got safely on to the boat. How we laughed at the thought of us, and all our colleagues aged 60 years or over, running and disrobing at the same time! I have to say at this point that my father was 83 years old and fit as a flea! I was the youngest member of the group. However, I had suffered a viral chest infection prior to the holiday, and I was the one wheezing and coughing. My dad was skipping along like a mountain goat, helping all the other 'elderly people' (most of whom were considerably younger than him) and thoroughly enjoying every minute!

Sadly, despite many jungle outings, we did not see a tiger, just a paw print!

We returned from this wonderful holiday and my family asked what had happened to my father, because he looked 10 years younger. (They didn't make any such comment about me!) The next few months were spent regaling others with our adventure, and planning the next trip, in 2006. By the end of the year, the second trip was booked and paid for. A slightly different one this time, but still with the aim of seeing a tiger! Sadly, it was not to be. My wonderful father, who had been so fit and healthy, became ill two weeks after Christmas. He was diagnosed with mesothelioma (a malignant disease caused by exposure to asbestos). After a stay in hospital to drain the fluid off his chest, he returned home and, very typical of the way he had always been, he tried to be as independent as possible. Sadly, he was so short of breath that many of his activities had to be curtailed. He could no longer walk his dog, and driving was out of the question. This was the opposite of how he wanted to be, and I knew in my heart that his illness would not last long because he couldn't bear the thought of becoming an invalid. Although none of us wanted him to die, we all knew that it would be better for it to happen sooner rather than later – before he became so ill that he was unable to do anything for himself.

Up until the day he died, my father remained 'in charge.' He even managed to get to the hospital to be marked up for a course of radiotherapy the day before he died (albeit with a cortege of helpers and a cylinder of oxygen!).

The night before he died, my mother suggested that she should stay with him, but he insisted that he was OK and that she must go to bed. The next morning, he asked my mother for a cup of tea, which he insisted on holding himself. He was very weak by then and, as my mother later described, he started to shake and the tea spilled on to his chest. Minutes later he died. For a long time my mother has felt guilty (and maybe even still does) about not staying with him overnight, and about allowing him to hold a hot cup of tea on his own. However, I believe that my father knew exactly what he was doing and exactly what he wanted, because that was the way he had always lived. I often tell my mother that my dad died as he had lived – independent, in charge and determined right up to the end!

As I said earlier, my father had a wonderful sense of adventure. Just before he died, he said to me, 'Well, love, I'm off on a different adventure this time.' I remember those words with such comfort, and often quote them to others who are facing bereavement.

When I finish this book, I plan to return to Nepal with my husband on the same trip as that which my father and I made, or a similar one.

And Dad – I am determined to see a tiger!

CHAPTER 1

Introduction

When we think of the term 'care home', we usually associate it with the elderly. Equally, when we talk about 'life-limiting illnesses' and 'palliative care' in care homes, these terms are mostly associated with the elderly. However, increasing numbers of younger people are being cared for in this type of environment, especially those with physical disability and learning disability, and some of these individuals have illnesses that require palliative care. Therefore all carers who work in care homes should be aware of the meaning of palliative care, and of all the different aspects that contribute to the provision of palliative care.

Carers often struggle when looking after a patient who is suffering from a life-limiting illness or a patient who is clearly going to die soon. They may feel uncertain about talking to that person about their illness, fearing that they won't understand, or that the truth would be upsetting to them. They may be frightened about the emotions that could surface when talking to patients and their families about cancer and other illnesses.

Some carers have difficulty talking about serious illness to one another, especially if that illness is cancer. The word 'cancer' seems to scare many people more than some of the other life-limiting illnesses that can cause similar symptoms and debility. However, not talking often causes more fear and distrust and makes caring very difficult for all involved. There is also a danger of creating a 'conspiracy of silence', where professionals, family and friends all know about the illness and impending death, but will not talk about it in the presence of the patient or each other. It may seem that by not talking about it, each is protecting the other from unnecessary distress. However, just because someone – whether they are the patient or the carer – is not talking about the illness doesn't mean that they aren't thinking about it. And not being able to voice concerns will ultimately lead to escalating confusion and distress for all concerned.

I have often heard carers say, 'Surely he would be better off in a hospice where they give proper palliative care.' Of course hospices do provide excellent palliative care, but they do not have the capacity to provide care for everyone with a life-limiting illness. This is why it is so important that the principles and practices of palliative care are taught, understood and used in hospitals and community settings such as care homes. If you ask most people where they want to be cared for in the last months or weeks of life, the majority of them would say in their own home. For many elderly people in particular, the care home *is* their home and this is where they want to stay and be cared for.

People are living longer and longer, and as they get older they tend to suffer from multiple and chronic illnesses. Consequently, the care that they require becomes more complex. Regardless of how old a person is, they have a right to be treated with the same care and compassion that a younger person would receive. They have the right to be heard and to be able to make their own choices about their care. Sadly, however, this does not always happen.

If you are a carer reading this book, whether or not you are a trained nurse you are certainly not alone in feeling less than adequate at times. This is why I wrote this book – to help carers who work in care homes to feel valued and confident in providing palliative care for their patients. I fully appreciate that carers who work in care homes are often busy, having a million and one jobs to do. However, good palliative care need not be any more time consuming than the general care that you provide on a daily basis. Good palliative care is not about how *long* you take to provide care for the patient, but how *well* you provide that care.

Remember: Older people have a wealth of life experience, they each present in their own unique way, and they were young and able once. Hopefully, all of us will live to old age, and we will then want to be treated with dignity and respect. Taking all of this into consideration, you can see how care homes are in a unique and privileged position to provide palliative care for our older population.

CHAPTER 2

What is palliative care?

Working as a Macmillan nurse, it is second nature to me to use the words 'palliative care' when describing the type of nursing that I do. However, whereas people tend to understand the type of nursing that goes on in areas such as Accident and Emergency, intensive care, coronary care, etc., the meaning of palliative care still seems to be shrouded in mystery. Despite the fact that palliative care is now a recognised medical specialty, very few people actually understand what the term really means, and very few like to ask. People tend to either nod and look sad, or say things like 'It must be really hard looking after dying people all the time.' Many people think that palliative care is only given to patients with cancer, and that it can only be given in a hospice. Most think that it is only for people who are dying, or given when the doctors 'can do no more.' There are many medical programmes on television that show the general public what goes on in a wide range of different nursing areas, such as Accident and Emergency, children's wards, maternity units, etc. However, very few programmes on palliative care are shown, and when such a programme is broadcast, it is usually accompanied by a warning saying that people may find viewing it upsetting. This reinforces people's opinion that palliative care is all about death and dying, when in actual fact it is more often about living with a life-limiting illness.

The actual term 'palliative' is derived from the Latin word *'palliare'*,[1] which means 'to cloak or cover.' I find this definition very helpful when I am trying to explain the meaning of palliative care. Put simply, palliative care aims to put a 'cloak' or 'cover' over a life-limiting illness. It cannot alter the progression of the disease, but it can alter the patient's experience of the disease by treating any associated symptoms in order to reduce discomfort. Palliative care meets the needs of patients with life-limiting diseases, whether or not they continue to pursue active medical treatment.

It is important to acknowledge that there is a difference between the meaning of the words 'palliative' and 'terminal', and that people who are receiving palliative care are not always terminally ill or dying.

'Terminal illness'[2] is a medical term used to describe an active and malignant disease that cannot be cured or adequately treated, and that is reasonably expected to result in the death of the patient. This term is more commonly used for progressive diseases, such as cancer or advanced heart disease, than for trauma. Whereas palliative care helps at all stages of illness, from the initial diagnosis of a life-limiting illness, terminal care usually relates to the last few days of life, when it is apparent that the patient is deteriorating and is showing symptoms of the dying process (*see* Chapter 18).

The definition of palliative care has many different versions – some short, some long – but they all use more or less the same language. The following two definitions are perhaps the most often quoted:

The National Institute for Clinical Excellence (NICE) defines palliative care as:

> The active holistic care of patients with advanced progressive illness. Management of pain and other symptoms and provision of psychological, social and spiritual support is paramount. The goal of palliative care is achievement of the best quality of life for patients and their families. Many aspects of palliative care are also applicable earlier in the course of the illness in conjunction with other treatments.[3]

The World Health Organization (WHO) defines palliative care as follows:

> Palliative care is an approach that improves the quality of life of patients and their families facing the problems associated with life-threatening illness, through the prevention and relief of suffering by means of early identification and impeccable assessment and treatment of pain and other problems, physical, psychosocial and spiritual. Palliative care aims to:
> - provide relief from pain and other distressing symptoms
> - affirm life, and regard dying as a normal process
> - intend neither to hasten nor postpone death
> - integrate the psychological and spiritual aspects of patient care
> - offer a support system to help patients live as actively as possible until death
> - offer a support system to help the family cope during the patient's illness and in their own bereavement

- use a team approach to address the needs of patients and their families, including bereavement counselling, if indicated
- enhance quality of life, and may also positively influence the course of illness
- be applicable early in the course of illness, in conjunction with other therapies that are intended to prolong life, such as chemotherapy or radiation therapy, and includes those investigations needed to better understand and manage distressing clinical complications.[4]

There are two acknowledged levels of palliative care, namely specialist palliative care and general palliative care (sometimes known as supportive palliative care or the palliative care approach).

Specialist palliative care is provided by people who specialise in palliative care, such as Macmillan nurses and the nurses and doctors who work in hospices. For these individuals, palliative care is the sole component of their role. Specialist palliative care is not needed for every patient who has a life-limiting illness, but should be available to anyone who has complex palliative care needs, such as unrelieved symptoms, complex psychological issues, or acute medical problems associated with their disease. Doctors and nurses who specialise in palliative care provide:

➤ clinical input – assessing the needs of the patient and suggesting treatment options
➤ education and training for other professionals
➤ advice and support for all carers involved in giving palliative care
➤ hospice inpatient care and/or day care facilities where necessary.

General palliative care is provided by all the usual carers, such as the staff who work in care homes, or district nurses who work in the community. For these individuals, palliative care is only one component of their nursing role. Carers who give general palliative care need:

➤ an awareness of the principles and practice of palliative care
➤ to work within their own sphere of confidence and knowledge
➤ to know when and how to access help from the specialist palliative care services.

During my teaching sessions, I devised an aide-memoire based on a recognised definition of palliative care. As you can see, each statement begins with one of the letters that spell the word 'palliative.'

Palliative care is:

➤ Pain relief and relief of other distressing symptoms

➤ Affirming life while regarding dying as a normal process

➤ Looking after a person physically, socially, spiritually and emotionally

➤ Living with a life-limiting illness rather than dying from it

➤ Intending to neither hasten nor postpone death

➤ Applicable to all life-limiting illnesses, not just cancer

➤ Team approach to address the needs of patients and their carers

➤ Individualised care, remembering that everyone is different

➤ Valuing each person and their family

➤ Enhancing quality of life for however long may be left.

Remember: Anyone who provides care can give general palliative care. It is the responsibility of every healthcare professional to ensure the provision of palliative care when it is needed. It is the right of every patient and their family to receive palliative care when it is needed. Such care is applicable and appropriate for all life-limiting conditions, in whatever setting.

There are many patients who have a life-limiting illness who never need input from a specialist palliative care service, but if you as a carer feel that someone for whom you are caring requires this specialist input, you need to know how to access it.

REFERENCES

1 http://en.wikipedia.org/wiki/Palliative_care (accessed 9/7/2008).
2 http://en.wikipedia.org/wiki/terminal_illness (accessed 9/7/2008).
3 www.ncpc.org.uk/palliative-care.html (accessed 9/7/2008).
4 www.who.int/cancer/palliative/definition/en (accessed 9/7/2008).

CHAPTER 3

What is a Macmillan nurse?

A Macmillan nurse is a trained nurse (registered nurse) who specialises in palliative care. He or she provides support and information to patients and/ or their carers who are affected by a life-limiting illness, such as cancer. Some people become very anxious if a Macmillan nurse is asked to visit them, because they believe that these nurses only visit people when they are dying. However, this is not always the case. A Macmillan nurse may see a patient when he or she is first diagnosed just to introduce themselves and the service and to provide any helpful information that is needed at that time. The Macmillan nurse may visit to help with control of symptoms, such as pain or nausea, at any stage in the illness from diagnosis onwards. Often patients live very comfortably within the limitations of their illness for weeks, months or even years between Macmillan visits. Equally, a Macmillan nurse will help to provide support if necessary when death is imminent. However, many patients die peacefully and comfortably with care and support from their usual carers, and do not require input from the Macmillan service at the end.

Although the Macmillan service is historically linked with cancer, Macmillan nurses now help patients who are suffering from a wide range of other life-limiting diseases.

They provide specialist palliative care for those patients who have complex needs. They do not see everyone who has a life-limiting illness, as this would be an impossible task. Many patients do not need the specialist palliative care that is provided by Macmillan nurses, as they are very well supported by all their usual carers, such as the district nurse, and carers who work in care homes and provide general palliative care. (Specialist palliative care and general palliative care are defined in the previous chapter.) Although in most areas anyone can refer a patient to the Macmillan service, referrals generally come from professionals such as district nurses, carers who work in care homes, consultants and general practitioners.

HOW DID THE MACMILLAN NURSING SERVICE COME ABOUT?

In 1911, a young man called Douglas Macmillan watched his father die of cancer. Distressed at watching his father suffer, he decided to do something to help others. He wanted people suffering from cancer, and those caring for them, to be able to access advice and information, so he founded the Society for the Prevention and Relief of Cancer. In 1924 this society became a Benevolent Society and changed its name to the National Society for Cancer Relief, providing practical help for patients and their families. The first Macmillan nurse was funded by the charity in 1975. Over the years, increasing numbers of nurses have been funded, and there are now over 2900 Macmillan nurses across the UK. Over the years, the name of the charity has changed several times, and it is now officially known as Macmillan Cancer Support (MCS).[1]

Although Macmillan nurses are often initially funded by the charity, they are mostly employed by the NHS. As with other services in the NHS, Macmillan services are free.

WHERE DO MACMILLAN NURSES WORK?

➤ **Community.** The majority of Macmillan nurses work in the community, visiting people in their own homes. These Macmillan nurses have overall knowledge of and expertise in most cancers and other life-limiting illnesses. They will usually make a detailed assessment during the first visit, spending up to an hour in the home. Depending on the situation and the wishes of the patient and carer, a further visit may or may not be arranged. However, the patient will always be given contact details to enable them to get in touch should they need further support. Usually the Macmillan nurse will inform the district nurse (if they are not already involved), and will also contact the patient's general practitioner.

➤ **Hospital.** Many hospitals employ one or more Macmillan nurses to provide specialist palliative care for patients on their wards. Like their colleagues in the community, these nurses also have an overall knowledge of and expertise in most cancers and other life-limiting illnesses. Hospital Macmillan nurses also give advice and support to the nurses and doctors who are caring for these patients.

➤ **Site-specific Macmillan nurses.** These nurses are usually based in hospitals. They specialise in providing care for people who have a specific cancer (e.g. cancer of the breast, colon, prostate, head and neck, etc.), and they have a high level of knowledge about the particular disease in which they have specialised. They communicate closely with the consultants involved in the patient's care.

➤ **Care homes.** Some Macmillan nurses are employed specifically to help to support patients and carers in care homes. Like their community- and hospital-based colleagues, they have an overall knowledge of and expertise in most cancers and other life-limiting illnesses. These nurses generally provide clinical and educational support, visiting patients when there is a need for this, and teaching the principles and practice of palliative care to the carers. They also communicate closely with the patient's general practitioner. District nurses also help to support patients who are staying in residential (non-nursing) homes, but in general they do not provide input for patients who are residing in nursing homes.

In addition to Macmillan nurses, there are other professionals who carry the Macmillan title, such as Macmillan consultants, Macmillan social workers, Macmillan dietitians, Macmillan GP facilitators, Macmillan radiographers, Macmillan occupational therapists, Macmillan physiotherapists and Macmillan lecturers. However, the availability of these services varies according to need and resources across the country.

WHAT HOURS DO MACMILLAN NURSES WORK?

Macmillan nurses generally work from Monday to Friday, 9 am to 5 pm, although many do now provide an out-of-hours service. Macmillan nurses are not an emergency service, and generally do not have the capacity to respond to a palliative care referral immediately. They respond to referrals by prioritising need, and it may therefore be several days before a Macmillan nurse can visit a patient. However, they will usually have made contact with the referrer and/ or the patient to assess how soon a visit needs to be offered. All Macmillan nurses provide specialist palliative care support and advice when needed, and will discharge patients when that need has been met. If further input is required, the patient can be re-referred and the Macmillan nurse will contact them to arrange further follow-up. Some patients are supported continually all the way through their illness until their death. Others may have periodic need only, and between periods of specialist palliative care support they will be able to get on with their lives.

HOW DO I REQUEST A MACMILLAN NURSE?

Anyone can ask to be referred to the Macmillan service, although usually this referral is made by a healthcare professional such as a district nurse or a doctor. Each area has its own referral criteria and referral form, but generally the reason for the referral should be clearly stated and an idea of the urgency of the contact identified on the form. Reasons for referral may include any of the following:

➤ advice on symptom control
➤ facilitation of communication and psychological support for the patient and/or their carer
➤ provision of information about the treatments and services that are available.

Once specialist palliative care input is no longer needed, the patient and/or carer will usually be discharged. Some of the reasons for discharge are listed below:

➤ the patient has died
➤ the patient or carer has discharged him- or herself
➤ the patient or carer has moved out of the area
➤ the problem that existed at the time of referral has been resolved.

Of course, re-referral is always possible if problems recur, and the patient and/or carer will be given contact details so that they can get back in touch with the Macmillan service if necessary.

Macmillan nurses do:

➤ have a greater knowledge of symptom control and the drugs that can help with this
➤ provide emotional support for patients and carers when needed
➤ provide palliative care education for other professionals
➤ work as part of the larger team, communicating with other healthcare professionals who are involved in the patient's care.

Macmillan nurses don't:

➤ take over the patient's care – the latter is provided by the patient's usual carers. In the community, care will be coordinated by the district nurse. In hospitals and in care homes, care will usually be coordinated by the patient's named nurse
➤ sit with people when they are dying; Marie Curie nurses provide this type of service

➤ provide 'hands-on care' such as wound dressings; district nurses and care home nurses provide this type of care.

Remember: Macmillan nurses are not just concerned with death and dying. No matter where they work, their aim is the same – to provide specialist palliative care for those who need it, to help patients and their carers to make informed decisions about their treatment, and to help them to cope with problems such as the symptoms associated with treatment and disease.

REFERENCE

1 www.macmillan.org.uk/about_us/our_vision/our_history.aspx (accessed 28/9/2007)

CHAPTER 4

What is a hospice?

A hospice is like a 'mini hospital' which provides medical, nursing and emotional support for patients with illnesses that cannot be cured. As with palliative care, its purpose is to provide relief from pain and other distressing symptoms and to support patients and their carers before and during bereavement.

Hospice care is provided free of charge for patients who are being treated. The majority of hospices in the UK are run by the voluntary sector and are registered as 'nursing homes.' The government provides approximately one-third of the funding, and the rest is made up of charitable donations. This is why you will often see charity collection boxes for hospices, and read in the newspapers about fundraising events.

The most important point to make about hospices is that they are not just for people who are dying. Of course, people do die in hospices, as they do in hospitals and nursing homes, but the average stay in a hospice is usually only one to two weeks, according to individual need, after which many patients return to their own home or care home.

Hospices are not about doom and gloom, even though for many the very word 'hospice' conjures up images of death and dying. Because of this, people often feel scared about either going into a hospice themselves, or seeing a loved one admitted there. If the job falls on you to talk to a patient about accepting hospice care, it is important that you explain what the hospice is like and how it can help them. Most hospices will arrange a pre-visit for a patient and/or their carer. They also have pamphlets describing the services that they can provide. It is a good idea to familiarise yourself with your local hospice and to have a few pamphlets available in your care home. Why not go and visit the hospice yourself?

There are approximately 750 hospices scattered around the UK.[1] The size and provision of service vary, but the principle of care is the same. Some hospices are attached to hospitals, but most are separate units. A large proportion of hospices are inpatient units, usually combined with a day care service. The usual number of beds in a hospice ranges from approximately 10 to 30, so clearly their resources for providing inpatient care are limited. Most hospices have one- and two-bedded rooms that look out over attractive views. Visiting is usually more relaxed than in a hospital, although most hospices will have a 'quiet' period during which they discourage visitors so that patients can get uninterrupted rest. Hospices are staffed by specially trained nurses and doctors, helped greatly by numerous volunteers who provide services ranging from making the tea and flower arranging to clerical work and fundraising. In general, the ratio of nurses to patients is much higher than in hospitals and nursing homes.

Originally the term 'hospice' referred to a place of shelter and rest, offering 'hospitality' to weary travellers. In 1967, Dame Cicely Saunders first used the term to refer to a place for providing specialised care for dying patients, at St Christopher's Hospice in London.

Now hospices provide the care known as palliative care that helps to relieve pain and other symptoms experienced by people suffering from a life-limiting illness. The majority of patients who are cared for in a hospice will have a cancer diagnosis, but care is also provided for patients suffering from a wide range of other life-limiting illnesses for which hospice expertise can make a difference. Some hospices provide care for babies and children, while the majority take people from early adulthood through to old age. The three main facilities offered by hospices are day care, inpatient care and hospice-at-home care. Some hospices offer all of these services, whereas others may only offer one or two of them.

DAY CARE

The provision of hospice day care is an important supplement to care, enabling many patients to continue living at home, whether this is in their own home or in a care home. Day care services may include medical and nursing care, physiotherapy, spiritual support, occupational therapy, complementary therapies, hairdressing and chiropody, as well as a range of creative and social activities. Patients usually attend once or twice a week, depending on need. The day hospice provides lunch and refreshments and the opportunity for patients to interact with others in similar circumstances – or to sit quietly if this is their choice. There is usually a bed available if they wish to rest, and a quiet room for patients who want this. When a patient is referred to a hospice day centre, the nurse in charge will generally try to schedule the patient for a day when others in a similar age range or with similar interests attend.

Referral to a day hospice is usually accepted from a professional carer, and completion of a referral form is usually needed. Check the procedure with your local hospice. You need to be clear why you are referring the patient, as care issues are significantly different for someone living in their own home and someone living in a care home (see case study below).

INPATIENT CARE

There are three main reasons for admission for inpatient care:
- ➤ symptom control – providing relief from pain and other distressing symptoms
- ➤ respite care – short-term care to give carers a break
- ➤ terminal care – for patients who are in the very final stages of their illness.

For someone who is living in a care home, the option of respite care would not be required, and usually the terminal care phase can be managed in a care home if this is where the patient wants to be. However, if a patient who is being cared for in a care home has symptoms that require more complex palliative care, a period as an inpatient in the hospice can be requested.

THE REFERRAL PROCESS

Referral to a hospice is made by a trained professional, such as a Macmillan nurse or a GP. The person who is being referred usually has a confirmed diagnosis of incurable malignant disease (cancer) or other life-limiting disease, the symptoms of which are difficult to control in their current environment, whether this is their own home or a care home.

When I visit care homes and am asked the question 'How do I know whether someone needs specialist palliative care or needs to go into a hospice?', I tell them that if they feel they have done everything they can do at their level of experience and the patient is still suffering physically and/or emotionally, then that is the time to call in the specialist palliative care team. If you as a carer are in any doubt whatsoever, you can always phone the specialist palliative care team in your area for advice.

HOME CARE

Some hospices offer home care services, sometimes referred to as 'hospice at home', whereby nurses visit patients in their own homes for periods throughout the day and night in order to provide palliative care support. In care homes that provide nursing care, this service would seldom be applicable, but in care homes that provide personal care only, support from hospice at home can be accessed. This can often make all the difference between a patient being able to remain in the care home until they die, and ending up in hospital.

PHILOSOPHY OF HOSPICE CARE

All hospices will have their own philosophy of care, which is usually based on the following definition of hospice care as stated by the National Hospice and Palliative Care Organisation (NHPCO):[2]

> Hospice provides support and care for persons in the last phases of an incurable disease so that they may live as fully and as comfortably as possible. Hospice recognises that the dying process is a part of the normal process of living and focuses on enhancing the quality of remaining life. Hospice affirms life and neither hastens nor postpones death. Hospice exists in the hope and belief that through appropriate care, and the promotion of a caring community sensitive to their needs, that individuals and their families may be free to attain a degree of satisfaction in preparation for death. Hospice recognises that human growth and development can be a lifelong process. Hospice seeks to preserve and promote the inherent potential for growth within individuals and families during the last phase of life. Hospice offers palliative care for all individuals and their families without regard to age, gender, nationality, race, creed, sexual orientation, disability, diagnosis, availability of a primary caregiver, or ability to pay.
>
> Hospice programmes provide state-of-the-art palliative care and supportive services to individuals at the end of their lives, their family members and significant others, 24 hours a day, seven days a week, in both the home and facility-based care settings. Physical, social, spiritual and emotional care is provided by a clinically directed interdisciplinary team consisting of patients and their families, professionals and volunteers during the:
> - last stages of an illness
> - dying process; and
> - bereavement period.

CASE STUDY BILL – DAY CARE

Bill had been residing in a nursing home for 18 months. He was 49 years old but, as is typical of most care homes, the average age of the residents was around 80 years. Bill was discharged there from hospital following radiotherapy for a brain tumour with a very poor prognosis. His family and the professionals looking after him were fairly certain that he would die quite quickly. However, Bill did not die. He continued to recover over the next few weeks to the stage where he was mentally alert, but physically disabled due to both the high doses of steroids that he had received and the effect of his brain tumour. The nursing home staff were concerned that emotionally Bill was just waiting to die, and that physically he was just wasting away in bed. Although it was a very proactive care home, like most it had limited resources for providing the type of emotional support and stimulation that Bill needed. Following discussion with the doctor and the Macmillan nurse, Bill was referred to the local day hospice. Here he received physiotherapy to strengthen his weak limbs, counselling to help him emotionally, and nutritional advice to help him to lose some of the weight he had gained due to long-term treatment with steroids. Bill was able to interact with others in a similar age group to himself, which was very important to him, given the environment in which he was living. Although he continues to live with a life-limiting illness alongside an uncertain prognosis, the day hospice has been able to provide him with palliative care of a type that the nursing home could not have provided.

REFERENCES

1 Hospice Information. *Hospice and Palliative Care Directory.* London: Hospice Information; 2006.
2 www.nhpco.org/4a/pages/index.cfm?pageid=5308 (accessed 28/9/2008)

CHAPTER 5

What is cancer?

I am including a chapter on cancer in this book because cancer is the disease that is most commonly linked with the terms 'Macmillan nurse', 'palliative care' and 'hospice.' Most symptom control in palliative care relates to cancer. However, the principles of palliative care and symptom control that are synonymously linked to cancer can and should be used to help people who are suffering from other life-limiting illnesses.

Although cancer is a serious disease, it does not stand alone as the disease that is most likely to cause symptoms and hasten death. In the elderly in particular, many other life-limiting conditions can be just as debilitating and just as deserving of palliative care. Also, because the very word 'cancer' strikes fear in most people, the seriousness of other conditions, such as heart disease, Parkinson's disease, renal failure, etc., is often underestimated. However, whereas many carers understand the basic problems that may be associated with other life-limiting illnesses, when it comes to cancer there is often much confusion and uncertainty surrounding the diagnosis, treatment and symptoms. This confusion only adds fuel to the fear that is manifested when the word 'cancer' is mentioned.

Therefore in this section of the book I shall explain some of the facts about cancer that I feel will increase your understanding, dispel some myths and hopefully alleviate some of the fears associated with this disease.

It may surprise you to know that there are over 200 different types of cancer, and there are over 60 different organs in the body where a cancer can grow. It may not surprise you that cancer is primarily a disease of the elderly. Understandably, the older people get, the more likely they are to suffer from damage to their body cells.

The word 'cancer' is derived from an ancient Greek word meaning 'crab.' The Greeks thought that clusters of cancer cells looked like the legs of a crab!

The term 'tumour' or 'lump' is often linked to cancer. However, tumours are not always malignant. They can also be benign, which means that they do not spread. The word 'cancer' only applies to malignant tumours.

Cancer is a disease of the cells which are the structural units of which our bodies are composed. All of the functions that are needed for life take place inside cells. We all begin life as a single cell in our mother's womb, and that single cell goes on to divide and multiply countless times. There are 200 different types of cell – as many as there are types of cancer – and they all do different jobs, have different shapes and behave differently. Normally, cells behave in an orderly fashion. Cancer is caused by cells that multiply in a disorderly fashion.

Cancer can develop in just about any type of cell in the body, so there is almost always more than one type of cancer that can develop in any one organ. Often, however, one type of cancer will be much more common in a particular organ.

For example, in the lungs, there are flat, scale-like cells called squamous cells and gland cells called adenomatous cells. Thus it is possible to have a squamous-cell cancer of the lung and also adenocarcinoma of the lung.

The following list shows how the words that are used to describe the different types of cancer tell us exactly what type of cell the cancer originated from:[1]

➤ adeno- = gland
➤ chondro- = cartilage
➤ erythro- = red blood cell
➤ haemangio- = blood vessels
➤ hepato- = liver
➤ lipo- = fat
➤ lympho- = white blood cell
➤ melano- = pigment cell
➤ myelo- = bone marrow
➤ myo- = muscle
➤ osteo- = bone
➤ neuro- = nerve.

The most appropriate treatment is decided on the basis of the type of cancer, the part of the body where it started, and the type of cell that has become cancerous. The decision as to whether to start any treatment is always finally made by the patient, or by the family if the patient is unable to make a decision. In the elderly, the decision is often made either not to treat or to treat conservatively in order to minimise the risk of side-effects. This may be because the overall condition of the elderly person is too frail, or because they do not want to receive any treatment. Many elderly people choose not to have any treatment, seeing their diagnosis as a natural ending to their life.

TYPES OF TREATMENT

Surgery

Surgery is performed either to remove the tumour, or to reduce the bulk of the tumour. It is generally only undertaken if the cancer has not spread, and if the patient is fit enough to undergo the surgery. Sometimes surgery is performed to improve the patient's symptoms (e.g. giving a patient a colostomy to prevent the tumour from blocking the gut, or removing some tissue from a brain tumour, known as 'de-bulking', to reduce the symptoms caused by the tumour pressing on the brain). For elderly patients whose condition is extremely frail, surgery is sometimes not an option.

Radiotherapy

This uses high-energy X-rays to destroy cancer cells *in situ*. It is generally given in order to relieve symptoms and slow down growth of the tumour. Patients have to be able to sit or lie still while receiving radiotherapy. Although this is usually only for a few minutes at a time, it can be difficult for an elderly person, who may be more likely to feel uncomfortable or who may have some mental impairment. Also, some cancers require several radiotherapy treatments, which can be quite gruelling in terms of travelling perhaps considerable distances on a daily or weekly basis. Once a part of the body affected by cancer has been treated with radiotherapy (irradiated), this area cannot be treated again. Depending on the area that is being treated, sometimes the symptoms get worse before they get better. For example, a patient who is receiving radiotherapy for lung cancer may develop soreness when they swallow. This is because the radiotherapy rays have to pass through the chest area where the oesophagus (food pipe) is located, and some of the healthy cells of the oesophagus will be damaged. However, these damaged cells regenerate quite quickly, whereas the cancer cells that are being targeted by the radiotherapy die off. The side-effects of radiotherapy also depend on the area of the body where the treatment is given. The most usual side-effects are tiredness, and reddening of the skin at the site of treatment. Radiotherapy treatment is not effective immediately, and it usually takes between 10 days and 2 weeks before any benefit is seen.

Chemotherapy

This treatment uses anti-cancer drugs to destroy cancer cells. The most usual way of giving chemotherapy is intravenously (directly into a vein) via a drip. Chemotherapy administered in this way is usually given six times in three weekly cycles. However, chemotherapy can also be given orally in the form of a pill. Many people feel quite worried when chemotherapy is mentioned, as they imagine being sick and losing their hair. However, there are many different types of chemotherapy, and not all of them have troublesome side-effects. As with radiotherapy, the most usual side-effect is tiredness. If the type of chemotherapy that is being administered is likely to cause nausea and vomiting, anti-sickness drugs will be given alongside.

Hormonal therapy

This treatment involves the use of either tablets or implants (small pellets that are injected just under the skin) and is used to either block certain hormones, or to alter their levels in the body. Some cancers 'feed' off the hormones that are normally produced in the body, such as oestrogen (the sex hormone that controls the menstrual cycle in women) and testosterone (the sex hormone in men). The two types of cancer that are often treated with hormonal therapy are breast cancer in women and prostate cancer in men. There are few unpleasant side-effects from hormonal therapy, the commonest being 'flushing' and weight gain.

CAN CANCER BE CURED?

Quite a few cancers can be cured these days, especially if they are found early enough. However, many cancers, particularly in the elderly, are more 'chronic' in nature, being regarded more as long-term conditions as is the case with many other life-limiting illnesses.

The main reason why cancer can be difficult to cure is that it can spread to a different part of the body to that where it started. The cancer that forms initially is called the 'primary cancer.' If some of the cells from this cancer break away, they can travel to other parts of the body and start multiplying there. This is referred to as 'secondary cancer' or 'metastasis', often abbreviated to 'mets.' For example, you may see a diagnosis written as 'Ca lung with bone mets' (Ca is the common abbreviation for cancer).

There are three main ways in which a cancer can spread:

➤ local spread – to a nearby organ
➤ via the blood circulation
➤ via the lymphatic system.

Certain cancers have professionally recognised common areas of spread. For example, cancers of the digestive tract commonly spread to the liver, and cancers of the prostate and breast often spread to bone. It is therefore important that, if you are caring for someone with a primary cancer, you are familiar with the type of cancer they have and the signs and symptoms to look out for that may make you aware of possible spread or other complications.

HOW DOES CANCER KILL?

As with other life-limiting diseases, the way in which cancer results in death varies. It largely depends on the parts of the body that are affected and the overall condition of the patient. In the elderly in particular, other diseases are often present, such as a heart problems, hypertension, diabetes, etc. Therefore it might not in fact be the cancer that is the cause of death.

Remember:

➤ Many people carry on living with their cancer, often continuing to lead a relatively normal life for weeks, months or even years.

➤ Many cancer symptoms could just as easily be symptoms of other illnesses or conditions that are much more common. The fact that someone has a diagnosis of cancer does not mean that every ache and pain they feel is necessarily connected to their cancer. They are as likely as the rest of us to develop the occasional headache or backache. Remember that the elderly often have other illnesses, and that the cause of their discomfort may be due to some other ailment, such as arthritis.

➤ Pain is something that most people fear when they hear the word 'cancer', but pain is not always a problem, and many cancers do not cause a lot of discomfort. Many cancer patients never need to take strong painkillers such as morphine. However, pain is subjective and it is important not to generalise. For example, two people suffering from the same type of cancer will experience the symptoms differently. In general, elderly people in particular seem to require fewer painkillers. This may be because they don't complain, or because their metabolism is slower than that of younger people, so they may not need as much painkiller for it to be effective. However, it is important that elderly people are treated with the same level of awareness of potentially distressing symptoms as are younger patients.

➤ Cancer does not 'eat away at the body.' Some people may become very thin, but this is not because the cancer is 'eating the flesh.' Weight loss is a particularly common problem among people with cancer, and is usually the result of them being unable to maintain nutrition. Even if someone with cancer is eating really well, it will be difficult for them to put on weight. (The exceptions to this are some patients who may be taking hormones or steroids, and who are likely to gain weight because of this medication.)

➤ Cancer is not contagious, and there is absolutely no danger of contracting the disease as a result of being with a person who has cancer.

➤ Some people worry that when a person has surgery for cancer, the surgery can make the cancer spread. It is possible that during the operation the surgeon may find the cancer to be more widespread than was previously thought, but the operation itself cannot cause the cancer to spread.

REFERENCE

1 www.cancerbackup.org.uk/aboutcancer/whatiscancer/typesofcancer (accessed 5/10/2008)

CHAPTER 6

What is a syringe driver?

A syringe driver is a small battery-operated device that is used to administer medication subcutaneously (under the skin) when swallowing is a problem. Not all medication can be given this way, but there are a variety of drugs that can be used in a syringe driver to control symptoms such as pain, nausea, agitation and chest secretions.

I have intentionally not written about the setting up of a syringe driver, the types of drugs used or how to calculate the doses, as all of these things need to be taught professionally according to the policies and procedures in your area.

Figures 6.1 to 6.3 show the three syringe drivers that are currently most widely used in the community and in care homes. The two Graseby syringe drivers require the user to measure and then set the rate setting. The McKinley syringe pump is digital and calculates the rate setting without the need for measuring. However, all three work on the same principles.

1 Graseby MS 26 syringe driver (*see* Figure 6.1).
2 Graseby MS 16a syringe driver. Figure 6.2 shows the tube and the needle that attaches the syringe driver to the patient. The needle in the photo is inside its sheath but uncovered, it is approximately 2 cm in length, and the tube is approximately 96 cm in length.
3 McKinley T34 syringe pump (*see* Figure 6.3).

Many people believe that syringe drivers are only used for patients who are dying. However, this is not always the case. Although they are very often used at the end of life when the patient is too weak to swallow, syringe drivers can also be used long before the dying stage to control symptoms when other routes for administering medication cannot be used. They can be used either temporarily to control symptoms such as nausea during chemotherapy

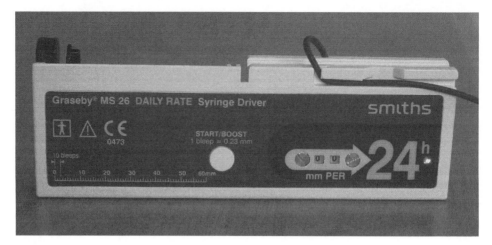

FIGURE 6.1: Graseby MS 26 syringe driver. (Image provided by Smith's Medical.)

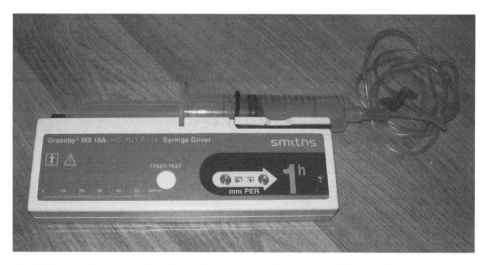

FIGURE 6.2: Graseby MS 16a syringe driver. (Image provided by Smith's Medical.)

treatment, or long term to control symptoms in the dying stage when the patient is too weak to swallow.

The two main routes for administering medication are the oral and rectal routes. In the UK, the rectal route (i.e. use of a suppository) is not used as often as in other countries, such as France. This has more to do with British preference than with the availability of drugs for use via this route. In the nursing home setting, elderly people in particular often don't like the thought

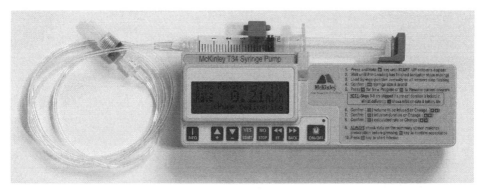

FIGURE 6.3: McKinley T34 syringe pump. (Image provided by CME McKinley UK Ltd.)

of medication being given in this way. Therefore, if taking medication orally becomes a problem, the syringe driver route may be more acceptable.

Problems taking medication orally may be due to any of the following:

➤ **Nausea and vomiting.** There are many reasons why a patient might be suffering from nausea and vomiting. If they are vomiting, clearly anything that is swallowed is going to be expelled before the body can absorb it. Furthermore, the patient is likely to be reluctant to take anything by mouth. However, it is important to remember that patients who are continually nauseated may be able to swallow and keep medication down, but absorption will be affected as gut motility will have slowed down. Therefore, even though the patient can swallow ant-sickness medication and keep it down, the likelihood is that it will not work because it is not being absorbed effectively. Carers could be forgiven for not recognising nausea alone as being a reason for setting up a syringe driver, as the patient is able to swallow and is not vomiting.

➤ **Difficulty in swallowing (dysphagia).** This may be caused by the illness itself (e.g. stroke, head and neck cancer, motor neurone disease), or by the side-effects of treatment (e.g. radiotherapy in the throat, neck or chest region, which can cause soreness and pain when swallowing).

➤ **Extreme weakness or a very sleepy patient.** This may be due to many factors, including general deterioration, side-effects of treatment, or the type of weariness that is seen in some frail elderly patients. The problem here is due to the frequent rousing of the patient to administer drugs, and the effort required to swallow them. All of this is extremely tiring for the patient, possibly at a time when they need to conserve their energy to do other things.

➤ **Taking large amounts of medication.** Although it is always preferable to take as few medications as possible, some patients may have to swallow a large number of tablets to treat various problems. It therefore might be preferable to convert some of this medication for syringe driver use in order to reduce the quantity that needs to be taken orally.

➤ **Poor alimentary absorption (inability to absorb drugs from the gastrointestinal tract).** This is not common, but can occur in certain illnesses and in prolonged nausea, as described above.

Once you know that a patient for whom you are caring needs to have their medication delivered in this way, you need to be able to explain to the patient, their family and other carers exactly what a syringe driver is, what it looks like, how it will be set up, and how it will help them.

HOW IS A SYRINGE DRIVER SET UP?

Syringe drivers are set up by a qualified nurse using medication prescribed by a doctor or a nurse prescriber. A written authorisation is usually needed from the prescriber, but the format of this will vary from one area to another. Some nursing homes have their own syringe drivers, while others borrow them from other sources such as the district nurse, specialist palliative care team or local hospice. The actual device weighs approximately 185 g (6.5 ounces). It is connected to the patient by a thin tube about 90 cm in length, with a small needle on the end (about 2 cm in length) that enters the patient at an angle of 45 degrees and is secured by a small transparent dressing. The needle is normally inserted at the top of the patient's arm, or in the upper chest wall, back of the shoulder or thigh. The medication in the syringe is usually changed every 24 hours (there are a few exceptions to this). However, the needle does not have to be re-sited every day, so long as the infusion is running to time and the skin around the site of the needle is not inflamed or sore. The syringe driver can be carried around quite easily in a specially adapted pouch, or in a pyjama pocket. If the patient is bed bound, the syringe driver can be placed under the pillow.

HOW WILL IT HELP?

The medication is absorbed slowly and evenly just below the skin surface. This avoids the 'peaks and troughs' commonly associated with some medication that is taken at intervals throughout the day. Because the stomach is bypassed, all of the associated swallowing problems described above will be avoided.

The drugs can easily be changed, added to or stopped, and the dose increased or decreased, according to the prescription and authorisation.

IS IT PAINFUL?

Insertion of the needle will cause a momentary scratching sensation, but once it is in place the patient should not feel any discomfort. Occasionally one of the drugs may cause irritation at the needle site, but this can usually be resolved easily.

CAN THE PATIENT EAT AND DRINK?

If they are able to and would like to eat and drink, there is no problem with this.

CAN THE PATIENT MOVE AROUND?

They can move around if they are mobile. The syringe driver can be easily carried in a pocket or a holster.

CAN THE PATIENT HAVE A BATH OR A SHOWER?

A shower would cause problems as the syringe driver must not be immersed in water. However, it is perfectly possible for the patient to have a bath with the syringe driver resting on a nearby dry surface.

ONCE THE SYRINGE DRIVER HAS BEEN SET UP, WILL THE PATIENT ALWAYS NEED IT?

They won't necessarily do so. If the patient is dying, the syringe driver will most probably remain in place until death occurs. However, if the syringe driver has been set up to control a particular symptom which then settles down, such as nausea, use of the syringe driver can be discontinued.

Remember:
➤ If the patient is swallowing normally and there is no reason for you to believe that there are any problems with absorption, the oral route should always be the preferred route for administering medication. If symptoms are not controlled when swallowing and absorption are not impaired, it is likely that the patient is either on the wrong dosage or the

wrong drug. This is not an indication for using a syringe driver, and you need to discuss the prescription with the patient's doctor or the palliative care specialist.

➤ When a syringe driver is first set up, it will take approximately three hours before the drugs begin to have any effect. Therefore it is always advisable to 'kick start' the patient's symptom control with an injection containing a proportion of the prescribed drugs at the same time as starting the syringe driver. Furthermore, any patient who is on a syringe driver may sometimes need an interval dose of one or more of the drugs in the syringe driver. The qualified nurse should liaise with the doctor to make sure that there are sufficient drugs available and that an authorisation is in place which allows that nurse to administer interval symptom relief when it is needed.

CASE STUDY MAUD – THE NEED FOR A SYRINGE DRIVER

Maud was a 73-year-old lady with lung cancer. Because of her general frailty and increasing breathlessness, she and her family made the decision that she should have no further active treatment, and she would move into a care home. I was asked to see Maud shortly after she arrived in the home, as she was very anxious about not being able to eat very much, and complaining of feeling nauseated. At the first visit, she was trying to eat her lunch with considerable difficulty. She said that she felt full after eating only a little food, and most of the time she felt nauseated, although she never actually vomited. She described this continual nausea as being her biggest problem, but was adamant that she did not want to go into hospital for any investigations or treatment. Discussion took place with her doctor to rationalise her medication and to stop all unnecessary drugs. Then we discussed which was the most appropriate oral anti-emetic (anti-sickness) drug to help with the type of nausea that Maud was describing. The anti-emetic chosen for her was metoclopramide, which it was hoped would improve her gut motility and prevent the feeling of fullness. Two days later I visited Maud to review her symptoms. She was no better, and her anxiety about not being able to eat was increasing. She was very tearful and depressed. Together with one of her trained carers, we described to her what a syringe driver is and explained how it would help. The most likely reason for Maud's continuing nausea, despite taking oral anti-emetic drugs, was that her stomach was not working properly and her gut motility was 'slowed down.' This was why she was feeling full after eating only a little, and also why the oral medication was not being absorbed properly. The use of a syringe driver would mean that the medication would be absorbed directly into her system. Maud was reassured that she would still be able to eat and drink and that hopefully she would feel more able to do so after a day or two. She was keen to give the syringe driver a try. The doctor prescribed the medication and signed the authorisation allowing the qualified nurses in the home to set up the syringe driver that same day. Within 48 hours, Maud was like a different person. Her nausea had settled completely, and she was able to eat and drink small amounts with enjoyment. Her anxiety decreased and she began to feel confident and supported in her new environment. Maud was told that when her tummy had had a good rest and when she felt ready, the nurses could try removing the syringe driver and she could go back to taking oral anti-emetics again.

CHAPTER 7

Symptom control

Although it is important to cover the topic of symptom control, I am only going to touch on the use of drugs when discussing each symptom. This is because I want this book to be read by as many levels of carers as possible, and I realise that not everyone will be a trained nurse. Also, it would take a complete book to comprehensively cover all of the medications that are used for symptom control in palliative care, and there are many palliative care books that concentrate solely on symptom control, and that are written by far more qualified people than me. (A range of suggested reading material can be found in the chapter on 'Further reading, useful websites and other resources'; *see* page 155.)

The only way that a patient's symptom(s) can be improved is by under-standing the cause and then applying the appropriate treatment. The challenge to carers is to continually review the patient in order to observe any change in their condition, so that the appropriate treatment can be implemented as soon as possible. People who are receiving palliative care have a life-limiting illness that is constantly progressing, which means that their condition can change quite suddenly. A patient may appear quite well one day and then seem very unwell the following day. Carers are in a unique position to observe the emergence of changing needs or symptoms, because they generally spend longer periods of time with the patient than do other members of the medical profession, such as doctors.

We use most of our senses when providing care for people, and with the right skills, carers can quickly detect unusual signs and symptoms.

➤ Using our eyes we can see such signs as broken skin, cuts, bruises, blood, and changes in the patient's ability to walk, speak or eat.

➤ Using our hands we can feel the patient's pulse, skin temperature, and any swelling, lumps or bumps under the skin.

➤ Using our ears we can hear breathing problems (e.g. wheezing or coughing), what the patient is telling us, and the tone of their voice.
➤ Using our noses we can smell body odours (e.g. urine infection, bad breath).

The symptoms of pain, fatigue, mouth problems, breathlessness, anorexia (difficulty with eating and drinking), constipation, and nausea and vomiting are discussed in more detail in separate chapters. The remaining symptoms are discussed in Chapter 15. I have tried to describe the following symptoms in a way that will be understood by any level of carer:
➤ pain
➤ fatigue
➤ mouth problems
➤ breathlessness
➤ anorexia (difficulty with eating and drinking)
➤ anxiety
➤ constipation
➤ cough
➤ dysphagia
➤ hiccups
➤ itching
➤ insomnia
➤ nausea and vomiting
➤ pressure sores
➤ restlessness and confusion
➤ sweating
➤ weakness.

Tables 7.1 and 7.2 show the percentage of common symptoms experienced in advanced cancer and during the last 48 hours of life. Table 7.1 was derived from several surveys, and is only intended as a rough guide. Table 7.2 is derived from a study of 200 hospice patients. Although Table 7.1 relates to advanced cancer, any of the symptoms listed could also be experienced by people with other life-limiting illnesses.

TABLE 7.1 Percentage of common symptoms experienced in advanced cancer

Weakness/fatigue	95%	Cough	30%
Pain	80%	Confusion	30%
Anorexia	80%	Pressure sore	30%
Constipation	65%	Pleural effusion	20%
Breathlessness	60%	Ascites	15%
Insomnia	60%	Bleeding	15%
Sweating	60%	Depression	10%
Oedema	60%	Drowsiness	10%
Dry/sore mouth	50%	Itch	5%
Nausea	50%	Diarrhoea	5%
Vomiting	40%	Fistula	1%
Anxiety	40%		

Source: Kaye P. *A–Z Pocket Book of Symptom Control.* Northampton: EPL Publications; 2005.

TABLE 7.2 Percentage of common symptoms experienced during the last 48 hours of life

Moist breathing	56%	Sweating	14%
Pain	51%	Nausea/vomiting	14%
Agitation	42%	Jerking/twitching	12%
Incontinence of urine	32%	'Plucking'	9%
Altered breathing/dyspnoea	22%	Confusion	9%
Urine retention	21%		

Source: Lichter I, Hunt E. The last 48 hours of life. *J Palliat Care.* 1990; **6:** 7–15.

CHAPTER 8

Breathlessness (dyspnoea)

Like pain, breathlessness is subjective – it feels like what the patient says it feels like. We all become breathless at times – for example, while running for a bus, competing in a race, or during a chest infection. Breathlessness like this has a reason and does not last long. However, in patients with a life-limiting illness, breathlessness often occurs with little or no exertion, and a person may become breathless even if they do not have an illness that affects their lungs, especially in the terminal stage of illness. Breathlessness can be very disabling and can have a severe impact on a patient's quality of life.

Being short of breath is not usually dangerous or harmful, and the patient will not 'just stop breathing', but it can be a very frightening experience, making the patient feel as if they will die due to lack of oxygen. For these patients, even the thought of going to sleep can be very frightening, just in case they stop breathing and don't wake up again. Breathlessness can also make activities of daily living very difficult. All of the activities that are normally taken for granted – even simple activities such as getting dressed or eating a meal – can become really challenging for someone who is struggling to breathe.

If you know that one of your patients is breathless, or is likely to become so, try to address the problem as soon as distress becomes apparent, rather than waiting until it is well established. For example, you could put an electric fan in the room, supply extra pillows, etc.

Breathlessness is nearly always accompanied by anxiety and fear, and this can make breathing even more laboured. You can help to relieve these fears for your patient by explaining what is happening if you can, and by reassuring them that they will continue to breathe. Always stay with someone who is acutely distressed about their breathing, as your very presence will be a reassurance.

There are many non-drug measures that can be very helpful when a patient is breathless, and that are very easy to implement in the home:

➤ Your presence – holding their hand or gently massaging their shoulders if this is tolerated is very reassuring.

➤ When you are not in the room, ensure that the call bell and anything else the patient may need are close by.

➤ Air movement near the face is very helpful and reassuring – for example, sitting by an open window or using an electric fan. A fan can be kept on a low setting overnight.

➤ Positioning is important. The most comfortable position is usually sitting upright with support, or leaning slightly forward with the arms resting on a pillow on a table. Lying flat usually makes breathing more difficult. However, the position chosen should always be the one that the patient finds most comfortable.

➤ Breathing exercises and relaxation techniques can be very helpful. A physiotherapist or specialist nurse can show you how to use these techniques.

➤ Help the patient with eating, as cutting up food, chewing and swallowing can be difficult for someone who is breathless. Try offering small frequent meals, and avoid giving foods that need to be cut up or that are difficult to chew.

➤ Help to reduce activities that make breathlessness worse. For example, you could help the patient with washing and dressing, and take them to the toilet in a wheelchair.

➤ An uncluttered environment will help to reduce any 'closed in' feeling.

➤ Encourage the patient to avoid wearing tight, restrictive clothing.

➤ Avoid asking questions that require lengthy answers, and encourage visitors to do the same.

➤ When patients are very anxious about catching their breath, they often forget to breathe out. Encourage them to take enough time to breathe out fully before taking in their next breath.

As mentioned previously, this book is not designed to give detailed information on medication. However, it is helpful if you are aware of some of the drugs that can be used to relieve breathlessness, especially morphine, as most people think that this drug is only used for pain relief. In smaller doses than are generally used for pain relief, morphine can be very effective in relieving breathlessness. It is often used in a liquid suspension that the patient can swallow. Other helpful medications include anxiolytics such as diazepam, lorazepam and midazolam. Oxygen is not always as helpful as people think it should be, given that breathing and oxygen generally go together. Very often in palliative care, the sensation of breathlessness is not caused by lack of oxygen, and the use of a mask or nasal cannulae can sometimes be a problem in itself. However, some patients do find oxygen helpful, even if the benefit is more psychological than physical.

Remember: Breathlessness is one of the most distressing symptoms in palliative care, and deserves your full attention to help to relieve it.

CASE STUDY BETH – BREATHLESSNESS

Beth was an elderly woman who was being cared for in a nursing home. She had end-stage heart failure, and her body and lungs were gradually becoming overloaded with fluid. Beth knew that she was dying and she had accepted this, knowing that her illness was incurable. She hoped that she would just 'go' in her sleep. She chose to have many of her medications stopped, as she was tired of taking such a large number of them. She just wanted to end her days peacefully, in as much comfort as possible, in the care home.

Beth's main problem was breathlessness. She was nursed in an adjustable bed that she could control herself when she wanted to change position. Although she felt ready to die, her greatest fear was of dying while 'gasping for breath.' Both the nurses in the home and myself had reassured her that this would not happen, and that we would work together to ensure that her fear was allayed as much as possible. The nurses provided an electric fan and arranged the room to be as uncluttered as possible. Beth's bell was pinned to her bed in a position where she could reach it at all times, and the carers were told that if she pressed her bell, they were to respond quickly. Beth was helped to choose small meals that were easy to eat, and was encouraged to sip supplement drinks throughout the day. Even though she declared that she could wash and dress herself, she was grateful for the help that was offered when she was feeling particularly breathless. Visitors were asked to be aware of the possibility of conversation exacerbating Beth's breathlessness, and they were often heard reading to her or playing music in her room. I liaised with her doctor about her medication, and with just a small dose of liquid morphine taken regularly, Beth found that her sensation of breathlessness eased considerably. We also obtained some pre-emptive medication and authorisation for the trained nurses to be able to give Beth an injection to relieve her symptoms if she started to panic or was unable to take her usual medications orally (*see* Chapter 22). Beth knew that everything was in place to help her if she should become anxious about her breathing, and because of this, she felt calm and less breathless. Over a period of several weeks she gradually became weaker, and she died very peacefully in her sleep, just as she had wished.

CHAPTER 9

Constipation

Constipation is a very uncomfortable condition that affects many people, but especially those suffering from life-limiting illnesses. Constipation is not so much about the frequency or infrequency of having a bowel movement, but more about the difficulty incurred in passing that motion. It is possible for a patient to have their bowels open every day and still be constipated if the stools are hard and difficult to pass. So long as the bowels move regularly and without discomfort, it doesn't matter if the patient only has a bowel movement once every two or three days.

Constipation is more common in the elderly because, as with other muscles in their body, the power of the bowel muscles diminishes with age. In addition, the elderly tend to take more medicines that have constipating side-effects, and to drink less fluids during the day.

The most likely reasons for a patient having constipation are:

1 related to treatment – for example:
➤ recent surgery
➤ some chemotherapy and radiotherapy
➤ medication – especially painkillers, such as morphine, but also other medications, such as antidepressants, diuretics (water tablets), non-steroidal anti-inflammatory drugs and anti-emetics (anti-sickness tablets)

2 related to debility – for example:
➤ weakness
➤ inactivity or bed rest
➤ poor nutrition
➤ poor fluid intake
➤ confusion
➤ inability to get to the toilet

3 related to the illness – for example:
➤ hypercalcaemia (high blood calcium levels caused by some cancers)
➤ disease related to the stomach/bowel area, such as a tumour
➤ spinal cord compression (a complication of some cancers)
➤ depression
➤ dehydration.

A patient who is constipated might complain of any or all of the following:
➤ stomach ache
➤ pain when opening their bowels
➤ feeling bloated and/or suffering from wind
➤ nausea and/or vomiting
➤ a feeling of incomplete emptying of the bowel.

If any of your patients are affected by any of the above, you need to be especially vigilant to prevent the constipation from getting worse.

There are many things that you can do to help to prevent constipation:
➤ If the patient is able to do so, encourage them to eat more fruit, vegetables and whole grains.
➤ Encourage them to drink more fluids.
➤ Allow sufficient time for the patient's bowels to be evacuated with comfort and dignity.
➤ If the doctor has prescribed laxatives, make sure that these are given regularly. It is always better to give laxatives regularly and to adjust the dose up or down for comfort, rather than give them on an 'ad-hoc' basis. For example, some people think that if they take a laxative, and are then able to open their bowels, they can stop taking the laxative until they 'can't go' again. However, this method does not allow the bowel to work efficiently.

If a patient is in the last days of life, so long as they are comfortable you don't need to worry about constipation. However, restlessness may indicate discomfort due to a full rectum, and this needs to be treated. This would usually be done with a suppository or enema.

If a patient for whom you are caring has loose watery motions, before you make the assumption that they have diarrhoea, ask a qualified person to check the patient's rectum, as this symptom can also be a sign of constipation. If the rectum becomes loaded with faeces that are too hard to pass, some of the liquid stool higher up may seep around the solid mass and pass out of the anus looking like diarrhoea.

I shall briefly mention bowel obstruction, as this is something that you may encounter, especially if you are caring for a patient with a cancer that affects their pelvic region, such as bowel or ovarian cancer. A bowel obstruction is a partial or complete blockage in the intestines that prevents wind, fluids or solids from passing through the system normally. The symptoms of bowel obstruction are usually described as a cramping abdominal pain, and a bloated feeling. There is commonly an absence of bowel motion or wind. Depending on where the obstruction occurs, associated vomiting may or may not be a problem initially. In some patients, surgery may be an option to relieve the blockage. However, in palliative care, sometimes active treatment is not an option and the symptoms must be managed with medication.

Remember:
➤ Any patient who is taking strong painkillers, such as morphine, will almost certainly need a laxative. The stronger the painkiller, the more laxative they will need.
➤ Ask your patient what their normal bowel habit was before they became ill. Some people are used to opening their bowels every other day, or twice a week, and so long as they feel comfortable, this is not constipation. However, if there is a significant change from their normal pattern, this could indicate a possible problem.
➤ Just because a patient is not eating, or is eating very little, this does not mean that they cannot be constipated. The bowel will continue to accumulate its own waste that needs to be eliminated from the body.
➤ Regular laxatives are usually needed, with adjustment of the dose as necessary.
➤ If a dying patient is restless, check to see whether a loaded rectum may be causing them discomfort.

CHAPTER 10

Fatigue

When we consider symptoms in palliative care, most of us would probably not think of fatigue, or if we did, it would probably be low down a list of other symptoms.

Fatigue literally means a feeling of being tired and lacking in energy. We all feel like this sometimes, especially when we are overworked, stressed or just generally run down – or indeed if we are trying to burn the candle at both ends! However, with this type of fatigue, the body is just letting us know that we are overdoing it, and we generally feel better after a good night's sleep.

Fatigue for patients with a life-limiting illness is experienced very differently. It doesn't go away after a good night's sleep, and patients often say that they feel just as tired when they wake up. Possibly the closest you can get to identifying with how it may feel is after a really bad illness, such as a bout of flu. Or you may remember a time you were in hospital recovering from surgery and wishing the visitors on either side of your bed would just go home so that you could get some rest. However, that type of fatigue is usually short-lived, unlike the fatigue experienced by the patients for whom we provide care.

Fatigue is the most common and troubling symptom for patients with life-limiting illnesses. However, it is seldom mentioned as a symptom, as it is not considered to be a 'proper' symptom, such as pain or vomiting. Doctors and carers don't always appreciate the severity of a constant feeling of fatigue, and often underestimate how much it can affect the patient's daily life. Unfortunately, there isn't a pill that can really help this symptom. Sometimes certain medications can help in the short term, but this often means 'another pill to take', and all medication has side-effects that may be more troubling than the fatigue.

HOW FATIGUE CAN AFFECT DAY-TO-DAY LIVING

Fatigue can be very frustrating. Tasks that we take for granted in everyday life, such as bathing, eating a meal or talking to other people, can seem overwhelmingly daunting to the patient. Constant fatigue is draining and can affect emotions and relationships with others. Some people may feel in low spirits and not want to bother with family or friends. Unlike other symptoms, fatigue can be very difficult for others to understand.

HOW CAN YOU AS A CARER HELP?

First, you need to understand some of the signs that may alert you to the fact that a patient for whom you are caring is suffering from fatigue. You may notice one or more of the following symptoms:

➤ reduced motivation and lack of interest in activities – for example, not wanting to join in the care home activities, and staying in their room

➤ lack of focus, short attention span and memory problems – for example, not being able to concentrate on reading a book or watching television

➤ sleep disturbances – for example, not being able to get off to sleep, or waking early

➤ complaining of their 'whole body' feeling weak or tired.

Remember: Some of these symptoms are common in many elderly people, but if the state of fatigue is a change from how that person normally is, you need to try and help. It is useful to mention any of the above symptoms to the doctor, as there may be a physical cause, such as anaemia (a low iron count in the blood), a chemical imbalance in the blood, dehydration, or the patient may be becoming depressed. All of these symptoms can be helped by medical intervention. However, if no physical reason for the fatigue can be found, there are many ways in which you as a carer can help to relieve some of the discomfort associated with chronic fatigue.

It is very important that you acknowledge the feeling of fatigue to your patient. Explain to them that you appreciate how frustrating it must be to feel so tired all the time, and that you will try to help them to find ways of coping with it. Just by empathising with them you can help to make them feel better.

Hygiene

It can make all the difference to how someone feels if they are not exhausted at the beginning of the day by major hygiene tasks. Instead of taking a bath or shower, maybe a wash in the patient's bed or chair would suffice. Consider helping them with dressing, especially pulling on stockings or tights.

Diet

Ensure that the patient's diet is as nutritious as possible, and that they are drinking enough. Remember that the very act of eating can be exhausting, so small portions should be served and the food should be presented in a form that is easy to eat (e.g. by cutting up the patient's meat for them).

Visitors

It can be very difficult for visitors to understand that their presence can be tiring for the patient, and you need to be tactful when discussing this with them. Suggest that they visit as often as before, but reduce the amount of time that they spend with their loved one. Explain that it is all right just to sit quietly with the patient, and that they don't have to engage in conversation throughout the visit. It is helpful to inform the patient who has arrived to visit them, and to ask them how long they want the visitor(s) to stay, or to tell visitors to report to a nurse before going in to visit, so that their presence can be monitored.

Sleep

Trying to ensure that the patient has a good night's sleep can help them to cope better the next day. Discourage the patient from drinking coffee or other stimulants before settling for the night, and offer them warm milky drinks instead. Review their bed and bedding in order to maximise comfort. Although this is not always possible in a care-home environment, try to keep noise to a minimum.

Naps

Encourage the patient to take naps throughout the day, especially while resting on their bed. Although it may seem to be a better option for the patient to be sitting in a chair, it is not always easy to rest well in a chair, and a couple of hours spent lying on their bed may make all the difference.

Reserving energy

If one of your patients or their family is planning a special occasion, such as a birthday celebration, or even an ordinary occasion, such as a hairdressing visit, it can help tremendously if they conserve their energy before the event by having a rest immediately before it, or a quiet day prior to and after a big event. Reassure the patient that if they are happy to go ahead with a tiring event, they will not do themselves any harm even if they do feel more tired for a while afterwards.

Remember: Although it is not always easy to recognise fatigue, and it is not easily treated with a pill, you as a carer can do many 'non-medical' things to help.

CHAPTER 11

Mouth problems

Mouth problems are very common in patients who are ill, especially when they are in the palliative phase of their illness. Sadly, however, the inspection and treatment of mouth problems is an area of nursing care that is often overlooked.

When we are healthy we tend to take basic functions such as eating, swallowing and talking for granted, but if you can remember a time when you have had something as simple as a mouth ulcer, it can make all those 'taken for granted' functions extremely painful and unpleasant. Having a cold can affect your smell and taste, reducing the pleasure of eating, affecting not only your appetite but also your overall sense of well-being. However, when the cold clears up, taste and smell return. Imagine what it must be like for someone who has lost their sense of taste altogether.

Fortunately, most mouth problems can be helped quite simply and effectively.

DRY MOUTH (XEROSTOMIA)

The most common mouth problem is a dry mouth (also known as xerostomia, pronounced zero-stow-meea). If the mouth is not being lubricated effectively by the patient's saliva, the mucosa of the mouth can easily become sore or infected. Chewing and swallowing food will be difficult, resulting in loss of pleasure in eating as well as poor nutritional intake. In addition, talking with a dry mouth is difficult, making the simple pleasure of communication uncomfortable. By treating a dry mouth, many other problems can be prevented.

Some of the causes of dry mouth include the following:
➤ side-effect of treatment, such as chemotherapy and radiotherapy
➤ side-effect of medication – most patients who are receiving palliative care

are taking drugs, many of which can cause a dry mouth; some of
the worst offenders are morphine, antidepressants and diuretics (water
pills)
➤ breathing through the mouth – for example, when a patient is suffering
from breathlessness
➤ poor fluid intake, due to not drinking enough, vomiting or having
diarrhoea; elderly people in particular often do not drink enough and
can easily become dehydrated.

If you are caring for someone who has any of the above, the chances are that
they will have a dry mouth.

MOUTH ULCERS

Mouth ulcers are small sores in the moist tissues inside the mouth and, despite
their size, they can be extremely painful. The cells that line the mouth are very
sensitive to damage caused by, for example, dentures rubbing or food trapped
under a denture. Mouth ulcers also occur in patients who are run down or
who are not eating properly.

TASTE CHANGES

Radiotherapy and some chemotherapy drugs can affect the taste buds. Dry
mouth, infections such as thrush, and general debility can also affect the sense
of taste. If a patient for whom you are caring complains of loss of taste, or of
taste changes (such as everything tasting the same, or being too salty, or too
sweet), you need to inspect their mouth to see whether they have a problem
that can be treated.

DENTURES

The majority of elderly people have full or partial dentures. Very often in
palliative care, these dentures become loose due to weight loss. In addition,
patients who are ill or bed bound will not be able to clean their own dentures.
It is impossible to eat and talk properly with ill-fitting dentures, and dirty
dentures will feel unpleasant for the patient.

THRUSH (CANDIDA)

It is important to observe the mouth carefully for signs of thrush. This is a very common problem in patients who are ill, especially those who are eating or drinking very little. In particular, anyone who is diabetic, on steroids or taking antibiotics will be especially prone to developing thrush. Sometimes it is very obvious that a patient has thrush, as you can see white patches on the inside of the mouth. However, in other cases there are no white patches, but the tongue may appear red and glossy. Another less obvious sign consists of sores at the corners of the mouth. Thrush can be very uncomfortable and debilitating, but it is easy to treat.

COATED TONGUE

Some patients may develop a very coated tongue. If you ask them to stick out their tongue, you can spot this easily.

You can help to ensure your patient's mouth comfort in the following ways:

➤ Every day, ask your patient how their mouth feels. Look inside their mouth and ask them to stick out their tongue. A small torch can be very helpful for this. Just this simple daily task can prevent problems from occurring or becoming worse.

➤ If the patient is able to do so, encourage them to clean their own teeth (or dentures) at least once a day. If they are too ill to do this, you will need to help them.

➤ Dentures should be cleaned thoroughly using a non-abrasive cleaner.

➤ When cleaning 'proper teeth', it can be more comfortable for the patient to use a small soft toothbrush, such as a child's toothbrush, and if you are cleaning the patient's teeth, a small toothbrush is less likely to cause gagging.

➤ Use vaseline or a flavoured lip balm to keep the patient's lips moist.

➤ Encourage the patient to drink fluids. If they are not eating or drinking normally, moisten the mouth at least every two hours using a foam mouth-care stick dipped in water.

➤ Milk, water, fruit or vegetable juices are the best drinks to choose, but any fluid is better than nothing.

➤ Avoid giving the patient citrus juices, or else dilute them with water (which will make them less acidic).

➤ Sucking ice chips will refresh the mouth and help to quench thirst.

➤ Fruit-flavoured ice lollies are very useful. If the patient is unable to hold and suck a lolly, it can be broken into small pieces on a saucer.

➤ Choose meals that are moist, and use gravies and sauces to make swallowing easier.

➤ If loss of taste or change in taste sensation is a problem, help your patient to choose foods that they can taste. Ask the kitchen staff to help.

➤ Eating pineapple can keep the mouth fresh and moist, but avoid giving the patient acidic fruits (e.g. oranges, grapefruit) if the mouth is sore.

➤ Saliva replacement gel can be very effective, and can be obtained on prescription.

➤ Chewing sugarless gum or sucking sweets can be helpful.

Remember:

➤ A sore, dry mouth can be very uncomfortable. In your care home, make sure that daily oral inspection is included as part of all other care.

➤ Tell the doctor or nurses immediately if you suspect that a patient has a mouth problem, so that treatment can be started straight away.

➤ Be especially alert to the possibility of a patient developing thrush if they are diabetic, taking a steroid drug such as dexamethasone, using inhalers to help their breathing, or taking antibiotics. Any of these can greatly increase the risk of developing thrush.

➤ Many elderly people, especially if they are ill, will lose weight. This will result in badly fitting dentures that will rub and cause problems.

➤ Nystatin solution is very often prescribed for patients with thrush. However, in order to be effective, it has to be swished over the affected areas in the mouth for at least one minute. Many weak or elderly patients may be unable to do this and therefore the medication will not be effective. If this is the case, discuss an alternative with your specialist nurse or doctor.

CHAPTER 12

Nausea and vomiting

Nausea and/or vomiting are very unpleasant symptoms that can occur in patients who have a life-limiting illness. Nausea is generally felt to be a more unpleasant symptom than actual vomiting, and is often described by patients as being just as distressing as pain, or more so. However, because the feeling of nausea is invisible, it is more easily overlooked by carers as a symptom.

There are a number of causes of nausea and vomiting, and consequently these symptoms can be difficult to control. Furthermore, choosing the right anti-emetic (anti-sickness) drug can be problematic, as each drug works on different receptors in the body to control different types of nausea and vomiting. Medical and/or specialist palliative care input is often needed to help to determine the cause and the correct treatment. In general, the only way to control these symptoms is by using medication, and very often this medication needs to be given via a syringe driver.

Some causes of nausea and/or vomiting include the following:

➤ **Chemical causes.** These are a common reason for nausea and/ or vomiting, and may be either metabolic (e.g. cancer-related hypercalcaemia) or drug induced (e.g. due to morphine).

➤ **Infections.** Examples include chest infection and urinary tract infection.

➤ **Gastric stasis.** Prolonged nausea causes gastric stasis, in which the gut motility slows down.

➤ **Raised intracranial pressure (ICP).** This can occur as a result of a lesion or tumour around the brain. Vomiting is nearly always a prominent symptom.

➤ **Movement-related causes.** Some patients may suffer from motion sickness if they are transported in a moving vehicle. Even the use of a hoist can bring on this type of nausea.

➤ **Regurgitation.** This is not quite the same as vomiting, and nausea may or may not be present. It is actually the 'spitting up' of food/fluid from the oesophagus or stomach. Regurgitation sometimes occurs for no apparent physical reason, but it can be due to disease.

➤ **Coughing.** Severe bouts of coughing can induce vomiting.
➤ **Constipation.** If food cannot pass normally through the system, it can result in a bloated feeling associated with nausea and/or actual vomiting.
➤ **Anxiety.** You will have heard of the expression 'sick with anxiety', and will perhaps have experienced feeling sick yourself when anxious about an exam result or job interview. If a patient is anxious, they may well experience associated nausea.

Careful assessment is required in order to help a patient who is suffering from nausea and/or vomiting. You need to find out from the patient whether there are any other associated symptoms. Look and listen in order to answer the following questions:

➤ Are they in pain?
➤ Do they feel sick?
➤ Does coughing induce vomiting?
➤ Do they have constipation or diarrhoea?
➤ What medication are they taking?
➤ Are they anxious?
➤ Is there any sign of infection?
➤ If they are sick, what does the vomit look like?

Although most patients with nausea and vomiting will require medication in some form or other, there are also many non-drug measures that you can use to help them.

➤ Minimise smells such as perfume, cooking smells, etc.
➤ Move the patient to a calm reassuring environment away from the sight and smell of food.
➤ Give the patient small snacks instead of large meals.
➤ Encourage them not to eat and drink at the same time – small sips of fluid can be taken to help to moisten the mouth, but drinking a quantity of fluid will fill up the stomach and hinder digestion.
➤ Pay attention to the patient's environment – make sure that bowls, tissues and fresh drinking water are always within reach. Fresh air is helpful.
➤ For patients who are unable to drink, attention to oral hygiene and regular mouth washes are important.
➤ Reduce movement, such as hoisting the patient or moving the bed.

➤ Ginger (e.g. ginger beer, ginger ale, crystallised ginger) can be very helpful if the patient likes the taste.
➤ Acupressure wrist bands help some patients.

As I have mentioned previously, this is not a medical book, and therefore detailed information about drugs and doses is not a feature of its content. However, because a wide range of different drugs are used to control nausea and vomiting, it may be helpful to be aware of what they are called and when they may be used.

Medications that can be used orally or via a syringe driver include the following:

➤ Metoclopramide (Maxolon) is a good drug to try if the patient has gastric stasis – that is, if they complain of feeling full and bloated, and food won't go down easily.
➤ Haloperidol is useful for feelings of nausea, especially drug-related nausea (e.g. when taking morphine).
➤ Cyclizine can be very helpful for movement-related nausea, and for vomiting due to raised intracranial pressure or bowel obstruction.
➤ Levomepromazine (Nozinan) is known as a broad-spectrum anti-emetic, and can be very useful if other anti-emetics have failed to help. It can be very sedating.

Remember: If a patient is nauseated, even if they are not actually vomiting, oral anti-emetics may not work as the person will have a degree of gastric stasis that will inhibit absorption of the drug into the body. This will also affect the absorption of any other drugs that the patient is taking in addition. In this case, it is nearly always necessary to give the medication via a syringe driver in order to bypass the stomach and ensure adequate absorption of the drug to control the symptoms. Once the nausea and/or vomiting has settled, the drugs can be administered by the oral route again.

CASE STUDY MIKE – NAUSEA RELATED TO TAKING MORPHINE

Mike was a patient in a residential home who had cancer of the lung. He was generally very uncomplaining, and most of the time he seemed very comfortable on his regular analgesic of paracetamol, and a laxative in case he became constipated. Although he did not have a big appetite, he enjoyed what he ate in small quantities. Over a period of about three weeks, he started to experience increasing pain in his chest area. The doctor switched his painkiller to something a little stronger, and this really helped for a few weeks. The next time that Mike's pain increased, the doctor decided to put him on morphine in a liquid format (Oramorph). Unfortunately, Mike started to feel very nauseated, and because he associated the morphine with feeling sick, he started to refuse to take his morphine. This soon led to a vicious circle, with Mike refusing his morphine and then experiencing more pain. The Macmillan nurse was asked for her help and advice by the manager of the home. At the first visit, Mike was very quick to say that he didn't want to take the morphine any more, but when it was explained to him how the morphine actually worked, and that patients sometimes did feel nauseated initially, he was willing to give it another try. The doctor agreed to prescribe haloperidol night and morning, which is a very effective drug for controlling morphine-related nausea. The doctor also took a blood sample for testing to check that Mike was not developing any other problems that might be causing his symptoms. Three days later, Mike was unfortunately still feeling very nauseated and he was also experiencing pain. He was becoming very miserable and fed up. It was explained to him that because he had been nauseated for some time, he was probably not absorbing the medication properly. He was shown a syringe driver and its use was explained to him. At first he was very reluctant to try this device, as he was mobile and he didn't like the thought of being attached to a machine. However, when he realised that he could still move around while 'attached' to the syringe driver, and that if all went well, after a few days when his symptoms settled, the driver could be discontinued, he agreed to give it a try. The doctor agreed to prescribe the medication, and the district nurses visited to set up the syringe driver (as the care home had non-nursing staff). It was decided to combine diamorphine (for pain relief) and haloperidol (for nausea) in the syringe driver. After three days on the syringe driver, Mike was feeling much better. His nausea had completely disappeared and he was no longer in pain. He was very keen to get rid of the 'machine', but he was persuaded to continue with the syringe driver containing diamorphine, while he tried the anti-emetics orally, just in case he needed them back in the syringe driver again. Fortunately, the nausea did not return, and Mike got through the next 24 hours without any problems. Two days later, the syringe driver was removed completely and Mike started to take the morphine orally again. One week later, when he was stable with no signs of pain or nausea, it was decided that he could stop taking the anti-sickness medication, but that the home should keep it in the drug cupboard 'just in case.' Mike continued to do well, with no return of his nausea, despite the fact that he was taking morphine regularly.

CHAPTER 13

Pain

When people think about life-limiting illnesses and dying, they often believe that pain is inevitable. However, not everyone who has a life-limiting illness such as cancer will necessarily experience pain. As has been stated often throughout this book, everyone is different, and therefore everyone's experience of illness will be different.

The word 'pain' comes from the Latin '*poena*' meaning punishment, a fine or a penalty,[1] and is defined by the International Association for the Study of Pain (IASP) as 'an unpleasant sensory and emotional experience associated with actual or potential tissue damage, or described in terms of such damage.'[2]

Pain is usually a sign that something is wrong – that there is illness or injury to the body. When there is damage to any part of the body, the nervous system sends a message along the nerves to the brain. When the brain receives these messages, pain is felt. Pain is generally divided into two categories.

➤ *Acute pain* has a relatively recent onset, and resolves as soon as the cause of the pain has been dealt with – for example, removal of the decayed tooth that is causing toothache, or removal of the inflamed appendix that is causing appendicitis.

➤ *Chronic pain* is pain or discomfort that continues for more than a month after an acute illness, or a reasonable time after healing is expected following an illness – for example, osteoarthritis (a degenerative joint disease that causes inflammation of the joints, and which is very common in the elderly), and recurrent backache following a back injury.

However, regardless of the definition of pain, the type of pain or how it occurs, the important thing to remember is that 'Pain is what the patient says hurts.'[3]

No two people will experience pain in quite the same way. What is described as excruciating by one may be described as bearable by someone else. Furthermore, a person's mood, morale and perception of the meaning of the pain can alter the way in which they experience pain and the severity with which they feel it.[3]

Think about the times when you have experienced pain and some of the things that have influenced or reduced its intensity. For example, a headache may be more pronounced if you are feeling in low spirits. On the other hand, if you are doing something enjoyable, you may not notice your headache so much. If you get toothache while you are at work, you may not feel it so intensely because you are distracted by everything that is going on around you. However, the same pain that wakes you up in the early hours of the morning may be felt much more intensely because that is all you have to think about. Another example is a pain that develops for no obvious reason. This type of pain will most probably be felt more intensely because you are scared of the possible cause. However, if you get toothache, you will be less worried because you know that the pain is caused by something wrong with that tooth.

So, with an understanding that pain is what the patient says it is, and that its severity can be influenced by other factors, how can you as a carer help to relieve a patient's pain? The important thing is to listen and observe. The elderly in particular can be quite stoical about pain, sometimes believing that one can't get old without discomfort, or they may be afraid to complain of pain in case they are sent to hospital for tests, or prescribed further medication.

Some doctors are concerned about prescribing pain medication for older patients because of their tendency to process medication more slowly than do younger adults, and because of side-effects such as constipation or mental impairment. However, when medication for pain is prescribed correctly, at the right dose, physical and mental functioning should be improved.

In elderly patients there is very often more than one source of pain. In addition to the possible symptoms from their life-limiting illness, the chances are that they will also have other conditions, such as osteoarthritis, osteoporosis (thinning of the bones) or some nerve damage (such as occurs in patients with long-term diabetes).

Never underestimate the discomfort that can be felt from a pressure sore, even a superficial one, or the discomfort felt by someone as they are lifted in a hoist or turned in a bed. Remember that their limbs and joints are not as supple as they would be in a younger patient, and may be stiff and painful to move after a while.

LISTEN AND OBSERVE

It is up to you as carers to report and document whether you consider that a patient for whom you are caring is in pain. The earlier someone receives treatment for their pain, the easier it is to get it under control. With the right treatment, it is possible to relieve all pain to some extent. The medication that is most effective for controlling pain will depend on what is causing it, and this is where the GP and/or specialist palliative care nurse can help.

When you are talking to a patient who has pain, it helps to find out as much as possible about how they are feeling.

➤ Ask them to describe their pain. They may use words such as 'throbbing', 'stabbing', 'burning', 'cramping', etc.

➤ Ask them where the pain is located. Is it in one place or does it spread around to other places?

➤ Ask them whether anything helps to relieve the pain or makes it worse, such as changing position, sitting down or walking, or heat or cold.

➤ Ask them whether the pain is there all the time, or if it comes and goes.

➤ Ask them what they think the cause of the pain might be.

Even if you are not a trained nurse, asking these simple questions will help you to explain the situation to others, so that a more experienced person can decide what might be causing the pain and the best way of treating it.

PAIN/DISTRESS TOOLS

Sometimes it is difficult for a person to describe their pain and distress. To monitor when pain or distress occurs, what it feels like, its severity, and what helps to relieve the pain, it can be very helpful to use a pain tool. There are many different tools on the market. Some of the simpler ones just use a number score. However, for a patient who has communication problems, such as dementia, a different approach to assessing pain or distress may be needed. Although I refer to each of the following as a 'pain tool or chart', any of them can also be used to measure distress.

Table 13.1 is a chart that helps the patient to select a word or words that best describe their pain. It is always preferable initially to ask the patient to describe their pain/distress using their own words. If they get stuck, you can use this chart to help them.

Table 13.2 is a simple number chart. The patient is asked to select a number between 0 and 4 that best describes the severity of their pain. This is a useful tool for obtaining a quick general idea of the severity of the pain/distress.

TABLE 13.1 Words that are used to describe pain

throbbing	pounding	shooting
pricking	stabbing	stinging
dull	sharp	pulling
gnawing	cramping	beating
smarting	sore	drilling
frightening	tiring	exhausting
constant	annoying	dreadful
comes and goes	agony	miserable
irritating	consuming	burning
discomfort	aching	excruciating
griping	blinding	twinges
torture	miserable	bruised

TABLE 13.2 Number pain chart

0	None
1	Mild pain
2	Moderate pain
3	Severe pain
4	Excruciating pain

The Wong–Baker FACES Pain Rating Scale (*see* Figure 13.1) uses faces to show a range of expressions that depict 'hurt.' It is used mainly for children, but can also be used for adults who have communication difficulties.[4]

The Abbey Pain Scale (*see* Figure 13.2) is an excellent tool used for patients with dementia or people who cannot verbalise.[5]

Pain is not only felt in the physical sense of the word. In palliative care in particular, we often talk about the concept of 'total pain' (*see* Figure 13.3).

Think of a time when you may have visited your GP with a symptom – say, for example, earache. The chances are that the doctor will examine your ear and prescribe you some eardrops or antibiotics. The GP generally does not have the time or the need to know whether the pain is affecting your sleep (physical), whether you are worried that the pain may indicate something more serious (spiritual), whether you are unable to join in your usual social activities with your friends (social), and whether you are frustrated because of loss of independence, due to needing people to care for you until you get better (emotional). This is what is known as *total pain*. However, you and your

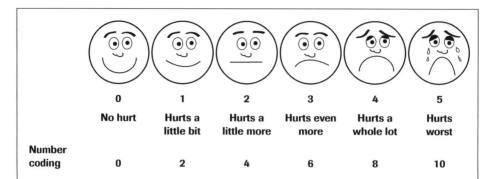

0	1	2	3	4	5
No hurt	Hurts a little bit	Hurts a little more	Hurts even more	Hurts a whole lot	Hurts worst

Number coding	0	2	4	6	8	10

Brief verbal instructions: Point to each face using the words to describe the pain intensity. Ask the patient to choose the face that best describes their own pain, and record the corresponding number.

Original instructions: Explain to the patient that each face is for a person who feels happy because he has no pain (or hurt), or who feels sad because he has some or a lot of pain. Face 0 is very happy because he doesn't hurt at all. Face 1 hurts just a little bit. Face 2 hurts a little more. Face 3 hurts even more. Face 4 hurts a whole lot. Face 5 hurts as much as you can imagine, although you don't have to be crying to feel this bad. Ask the patient to choose the face that best describes how they are feeling.

Complete the chart as in the example below:

Date	Time	Which face number	What helped
1/1/08	09.00	1	Making patient more comfortable by changing her position
	09.30	0	
1/1/08	12.00	4	Paracetamol 1 g given as prescribed
	12.30	1	
1/1/08	16.30	2	Helped back to bed and given 5 mg of oral morphine as prescribed
1/1/08	17.00	0	

FIGURE 13.1 Wong–Baker FACES Pain Rating Scale. Reproduced with the permission of the publisher from Hockenberry MJ, Wilson D and Winkelstein ML. *Wong's Essentials of Paediatric Nursing*, 7th edn. St Louis, MO: CV Mosby; 2005. p. 1259.

Abbey Pain Scale

For measurement of pain in people with dementia who cannot verbalise.

How to use scale: While observing the resident, score questions 1 to 6

Name of resident: ....

Name and designation of person completing the scale: ....

Date: ....**Time:** ....

Latest pain relief given was...**at** ....**hrs.**

Q1.	**Vocalisation** eg. whimpering, groaning, crying *Absent 0 Mild 1 Moderate 2 Severe 3*	**Q1** [ ]
Q2.	**Facial expression** eg: looking tense, frowning grimacing, looking frightened *Absent 0 Mild 1 Moderate 2 Severe 3*	**Q2** [ ]
Q3.	**Change in body language** eg: fidgeting, rocking, guarding part of body, withdrawn *Absent 0 Mild 1 Moderate 2 Severe 3*	**Q3** [ ]
Q4.	**Behavioural Change** eg: increased confusion, refusing to eat, alteration in usual patterns *Absent 0 Mild 1 Moderate 2 Severe 3*	**Q4** [ ]
Q5.	**Physiological change** eg: temperature, pulse or blood pressure outside normal limits, perspiring, flushing or pallor *Absent 0 Mild 1 Moderate 2 Severe 3*	**Q5** [ ]
Q6.	**Physical changes** eg: skin tears, pressure areas, arthritis, contractures, previous injuries. *Absent 0 Mild 1 Moderate 2 Severe 3*	**Q6** [ ]

Add scores for 1 – 6 and record here ⟹ Total Pain Score [ ]

Now tick the box that matches the Total Pain Score ⟹

0 – 2	3 – 7	8 – 13	14+
No pain	Mild	Moderate	Severe

Finally, tick the box which matches the type of pain ⟹

Chronic	Acute	Acute on Chronic

Abbey, J; De Bellis, A; Piller, N; Esterman, A; Giles, L; Parker, D and Lowcay, B.
Funded by the JH & JD Gunn Medical Research Foundation 1998 – 2002
(This document may be reproduced with this acknowledgment retained)

FIGURE 13.2: Abbey Pain Scale. Reproduced with permission. Available at www. dementiacareaustralia.com

Physical pain		Spiritual pain
Hurting		General fears
Not sleeping		Fear of dying
Not eating		Anxiety
Restless		General unrest
Mobility affected		Nightmares
	TOTAL PAIN	
Emotional pain		Social pain
Anger		Change of role
Frustration		Loss of finances
Despair		Loss of independence
Irritable with others		Helplessness
Mood swings		Worry about family/others

FIGURE 13.3 Total pain.

doctor are fairly certain that your pain and debility should only be transient, and that in a few days' time you should be back to normal. For someone with a life-limiting illness, total pain is likely to be more of an issue.

A DESCRIPTION OF TOTAL PAIN

Consider the following description of total pain for May, an elderly resident in a care home.

> May has been diagnosed with heart failure, and has been managing reasonably well until just recently, when she started to become more breathless and her hands and feet started to swell. The doctor has visited and prescribed a diuretic (water tablet) to reduce the swelling and ease May's breathing. She will probably have to remain on these tablets to prevent her symptoms from recurring. May has always enjoyed taking part in activities in the main lounge with some of the other residents, but now she feels breathless if she does too much (physical pain). She is worried about her deterioration and wonders whether the doctor has been honest with her or if there may be something he is not telling her (spiritual pain). She is very frustrated and embarrassed because

whereas previously she could always walk the short distance to the toilet and get there in time, she can no longer walk quickly enough, and because of the water tablets she finds that she wets herself before she can get there (emotional pain). May used to enjoy going out for Sunday lunch with her family, but she has stopped doing this because of her worries about not being close enough to the toilet (social pain).

So what can you do to help?

1 **Physical pain** – breathlessness. The GP has prescribed medication to relieve this, but there are also non-drug measures that you can use to help. Encourage May to take her time. Sitting in a more upright chair may be helpful. Sitting in the lounge near an open window, or near an electric fan, will help to increase air movement around her face. Encourage her family to bring in loose comfortable clothing (*see* Chapter 8).

2 **Spiritual pain** – worrying whether the doctor has told her everything. Allow time for May to express her fears. If you are able to do so, reiterate what the doctor said and offer explanations and reassurance. Ask the doctor to visit again to talk to May. Make sure that someone is with her when this happens so that they can also listen to what the doctor is saying.

3 **Social pain** – not being able to go out for lunch with her family. You could suggest that May's family share Sunday lunch with her in the home, or that they choose a restaurant that is not too far away, to keep the journey short, and that their table is close to a toilet.

4 **Emotional pain** – frustration and embarrassment due to loss of independence. Use any resources that help to maintain May's independence and ease her embarrassment, such as a commode in her room, sitting her near an exit for the nearest toilet, and using a wheelchair to get her to the toilet. Discuss whether she might be willing to use a small incontinence pad for extra security.

Pain can seriously affect an elderly person's enjoyment of life, and it should always be taken seriously.

Remember: Pain is what the patient says it is, and the right treatment is the one that relieves the pain.

REFERENCES

1 www.medterms.com/script/main/art.asp?articlekay=4723 (accessed 16/11/2007)
2 www.IASP-pain.org/am/template.cfm?section=pain-definition&template (accessed 16/11/2007)

3 Twycross R. *Symptom Management in Advanced Cancer.* 2nd edn. Oxford: Radcliffe Medical Press; 1997.

4 Hockenberry MJ, Wilson D, Winkelstein ML. *Wong's Essentials of Paediatric Nursing.* 7th edn. St Louis, MO: CV Mosby; 2005; www.mosbysdrugconsult.com/cgi-bin/forumregurgitatorcaller.pl (accessed 16/11/2007)

5 www.racgp.org.au/silverbookonline/4-6.asp-8k (accessed 16/11/2007)

CHAPTER 14

Difficulty with eating and drinking

Apart from the fact that we need food and fluid for our survival, the act of eating and drinking is also one of the most basic pleasures in life. Eating and drinking is a highly social activity that most of us engage in with our friends or family. Recall a time when you lost your appetite during a bout of illness, or when you were going through a period of stress. Remember how it felt not to be hungry, and how the people who cared for you tried to encourage you to eat. Encouraging someone who is ill to eat is one of the most basic acts of caring that we undertake, and if we cannot help that person to eat, for whatever reason, we may feel sad and inadequate. Equally, it can be very difficult for families, friends and carers to understand that as a patient becomes more ill, their appetite and their need for diet and fluids decrease. Helping with nutrition is an important part of caring for a patient, but so long as you have tried to help and encourage them with eating and drinking, you should not consider your care to have failed if you do not succeed. Some ways in which you can help the patient are described below.

If the patient is able to feed him- or herself:

➤ Ensure that any symptoms such as pain, nausea or constipation are dealt with, as these symptoms will have an effect on appetite.
➤ Ensure that good oral hygiene is being given and that the patient's dentures (if worn) fit properly.
➤ Talk to the patient about their dietary preferences and dislikes, and liaise with the kitchen staff to enlist their help.
➤ Ensure that meals are provided in small quantities at the right temperature and at regular intervals.
➤ Ensure that the patient is comfortable, able to reach their meal, and has the correct implements to use.
➤ If the patient is breathless, eating can be difficult (remember what it feels

like trying to eat with a blocked up nose when you have a cold). Eating suddenly becomes hard work! Aim to reduce the 'effort' of eating – for example, by cutting food into small pieces, and serving soft food that is easily swallowed, such as soups and puddings.

➤ If the patient is prone to feeling nauseated, removing the lids from plates of food can reduce the sudden surge of smell that can make the feeling of nausea worse.

➤ If you are caring for a patient who is having prescribed supplementary drinks – the kind that are usually supplied in small cartons – there are ways of making these more appetising. There can be nothing worse than drinking from a small carton that has been standing around in a warm room. Most people find these drinks more palatable if they are well chilled and presented in a glass or other drinking vessel.

➤ Some patients get on very well using a straw to suck up fluids. However, when a patient becomes very weak, the effort of sucking liquid up a straw may be too much for them. If this is the case, a small funneled beaker may be more helpful.

If the patient is no longer able to feed him- or herself, you can obviously help by spoon-feeding. However, be very sensitive to the fact that they may not want, or need, the food that you are offering, and that 'forcing' food and fluids on a patient who is nearing the end of life can cause distress and discomfort.

When a patient is entering the final stage of their life, eating and drinking often become more difficult. Some patients already have a percutaneous endo-scopic gastroscopy (PEG) feeding tube, so will continue to be nourished via this tube. However, for those patients without such access, family and friends can really struggle with the belief that their loved one is 'starving', and feel that they should be fed artificially – for example, by having an intravenous infusion (a drip) set up. In most care homes it is not possible to support a patient on intravenous fluids, as doctors are generally not readily available to re-site the needle when necessary. This means that the patient would have to go into hospital. Some care homes are equipped to provide subcutaneous fluids for patients who are considered to be very dehydrated. However, when a patient is nearing the end of life, artificial feeding is often more harmful than helpful. Families need to be reassured that, at this stage, their loved one will not 'die of starvation or dehydration', and that not eating and drinking towards the end of life is the body's natural way of preparing for death. Indeed, 'pushing' fluids into someone who is near the end of life can do more harm than good, as it can increase the strain on an already failing system. For example, respiratory secretions may be increased.

When a patient is entering the final stage of their life, they do not feel the type of thirst that we feel – which can only be quenched by drinking a glass of water. For them, the sensation of thirst is felt 'at mouth level', and they will feel relief from this if they have their mouth moistened. This can be done by offering small sips of water, or giving them small slivers of ice to suck. Ice lollies chopped into small pieces can also be very refreshing. If the patient is no longer able to manage swallowing or sucking, you can help to moisten their mouth by using foam swabs (or something similar) dipped in water, and applying a moisturising agent to their lips (*see* Chapter 11). This is something that you can encourage the family to do themselves, thus helping to give them a feeling of being needed and of doing something practical and comforting for the patient.

Remember:
➤ It is helpful to consult a dietitian for advice, although this is not necessary if the patient is imminently dying.
➤ Carers can become quite obsessed with weighing patients and trying to make sure that they eat a good diet. However, when someone is in the palliative stage of their life, the importance of nutrition should shift from food designed to provide the correct nutrients to food that the patient enjoys. No food should be withheld if it is something that the patient enjoys eating. Palliative care is not a time for diets, especially towards the end of life, and even diabetic patients should be able to enjoy a little of what they fancy.
➤ Cancer can affect the way in which the body metabolises protein, carbohydrates and fat. This means that no matter how much the person eats, weight loss will still occur.

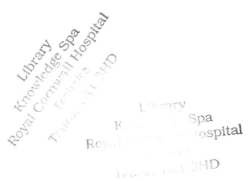

CHAPTER 15

Other symptoms

The following symptoms are ones that you may encounter when providing palliative care for a patient. Very often these symptoms need specialist palliative care or medical input, but there is nearly always something that you as a carer can do to help.

The important thing is for you to report what is happening and to communicate with others who are involved in caring for the patient.

ANXIETY

A patient may be anxious for many reasons, and the key to this distressing symptom is communication to try to find out the cause of the anxiety. If the source of the anxiety can be resolved – for example, by ensuring that the call bell is answered quickly, or leaving a light on overnight – this is the obvious 'treatment' to use. However, if the anxiety is long-standing, or due to factors that cannot easily be resolved, you will need to work with the patient to help to reduce their anxiety. This may involve setting aside time each day to talk through their fears, or calling in a specialist such as a counsellor. Often medication is needed to help to reduce the feeling of anxiety, but it should not take the place of human comfort. Sometimes extreme anxiety can be manifested as confusion.

CONFUSION/RESTLESSNESS

This is a common problem in patients who are receiving palliative care, especially in the elderly, and it can be a very difficult symptom for carers to deal with. Families tend to be distressed if their loved one becomes confused, as previous 'normal' behaviours and conversation can suddenly become quite bizarre. It is important to explain to the family that the confusion is due to the patient's illness, or to the treatment they are receiving, and that their loved one is not 'going mad.' Confusion in a patient who is receiving palliative care can be due to a number of factors, including the following:

➤ drug side-effects
➤ brain metastases (the spread of cancer to the brain)
➤ infection, especially in the elderly (e.g. infection of the chest or urinary tract)
➤ full bladder and/or rectum
➤ chemical imbalance (e.g. hypercalcaemia or uraemia)
➤ hypoxia (lack of oxygen) (e.g. in a patient who is very breathless).

Remember also that if the patient (especially if they are elderly) has been used to drinking alcohol, they may be suffering from withdrawal effects which can be manifested as confusion.

Very often the reason for the confusion can be identified and treated, and you need to discuss the matter with your palliative care specialist and/or the doctor. There are certain drugs that can be used. However, in addition to medication, there are many ways in which you as a carer can help.

➤ Provide the patient with a quiet environment, and avoid sudden noise.
➤ Use a gentle soothing approach, avoiding sudden movements.
➤ Talk to the patient – tell them who you are, what you are doing, what day it is, etc.
➤ Try to restrict the number of carers to two or three familiar faces.
➤ Close relatives may help to calm the patient.
➤ Familiar objects in the room are helpful – try not to move things around.
➤ Gentle background music may sometimes be helpful.
➤ Provide soft lighting.

Remember: Some, all or none of the above may be helpful, or some may even make the situation worse – it is very much a matter of trial and error.

In the last few days of life, 'terminal restlessness' is quite common, but very distressing to those watching. Sometimes there is an obvious reason, such as a full bladder or rectum. Very often, however, it is just a normal part of the dying process. Use any of the above approaches to help to soothe the patient, but always make sure that they have medication that is given early and in a timely fashion to help to avoid this problem, and to reduce the stress for carers and family.

COUGH

Cough is a reflex action that happens to everyone from time to time in order to clear secretions from their lungs. However, in a patient who is already weak due to illness, repetitive coughing can result in insomnia, exhaustion and vomiting, and it can also affect normal activities such as eating and talking. Cough can be due to any of the following:

➤ infection

➤ disease of the lungs

➤ build-up of fluid in the lungs, such as occurs in heart failure

➤ dysphagia (difficulty with swallowing).

Patients with a cough will often need medication, but you can also help to relieve the symptoms by assisting the patient into a sitting position, providing extra pillows, etc. Sometimes adding gentle steam to the atmosphere helps by moistening the air. Taking sips of fluid or sucking a sweet may help a tickly cough.

DYSPHAGIA (DIFFICULTY WITH SWALLOWING)

The commonest cause of dysphagia in patients with a life-limiting illness is disease of the oesophagus (food pipe), such as cancer. Dysphagia can also occur in patients who have suffered from a stroke, and in those with a neurological illness, such as motor neurone disease (MND). However, it is important to remember that discomfort in the mouth and throat (e.g. when a patient has thrush) will also result in discomfort when swallowing. A thorough assessment should always be undertaken for any patient who is suffering in this way, as in addition to the distress that dysphagia causes the patient, complications are very likely to occur, such as choking and inhalation pneumonia (infection of the lungs that can occur following inhalation of food particles). You should seek professional advice as soon as possible. This will usually result in the patient being assessed by a speech and language therapist, who will be able to advise on feeding techniques and the types and textures of food and fluid that can be given.

HICCUPS

If you have ever suffered from a bout of hiccups, you will know how irritating they can be, but they generally last for only a few minutes. For some patients, however, hiccups can be a real problem, either occurring in frequent bouts, or continuing without a break. They can be exhausting, and affect eating,

drinking and conversation. Hiccups may be due to any of the following:
➤ gastric distension (bloating due to wind)
➤ disease of the liver
➤ pressure on the phrenic nerve (the nerve that causes the hiccup reflex)
➤ uraemia (which occurs in kidney failure, when urea and other waste
   products that are normally excreted into the urine are instead retained in
   the blood).

If a patient for whom you are caring has bouts of hiccups or continuous
hiccups, don't pass it off as a minor symptom, as it can be really distressing to
someone who is ill. There are many 'old wives' tales' about cures for hiccups.
Most of these remedies are based on distraction or concentration, such as
drinking from the opposite side of a glass. Breathing in and out of a paper bag
can be effective by causing a change in the ratio of oxygen to carbon dioxide
levels in the blood. However, for patients with relentless hiccups, it is likely
that medication will be needed to help to relieve this symptom.

ITCHING

Like sweating and hiccups, for the majority of us itching is quite a trivial
symptom and easily remedied. A normal itch is something that happens to
most of us quite often, and a scratch is usually all that is needed to relieve it.
However, itching that continues incessantly can be very distressing and can
severely disrupt sleep. Constant itching occurs for a reason, and in a patient
who is receiving palliative care, the most likely reasons are drug side-effects, or
a direct result of their illness. You need to alert your palliative care specialist
or the patient's doctor, as medication and/or other treatment can very often
be helpful. You can also help by:
➤ treating dry skin using bath emollients rather than soaps, and aqueous
   creams
➤ encouraging the patient not to eat spicy foods
➤ avoiding hot rooms and hot baths
➤ ensuring that the patient wears soft clothing made of natural fabrics
➤ skin-cooling techniques (*see* 'Sweating' section below).

INSOMNIA (SLEEPLESSNESS)

Sleep is as essential as food, air and water. We need sleep to be able to function properly. When people are ill, they need sleep even more to help their
body to recover if that is possible, and if recovery is not possible, they certainly

need good-quality sleep to help them to cope with each day. You will no doubt have experienced nights when you cannot sleep, or when you felt that you had been awake for most of the night. This will have an impact on the next day, making you feel tired and less able to cope. Insomnia can be very distressing, frustrating and exhausting. If a patient for whom you are caring is having sleepless nights, you need to be aware of this so that you can help them. Often a patient can appear to have had a good night's sleep, and you might be surprised if they tell you that they haven't slept very well. However, it is the way that they perceive their quality of sleep that is important, and if they say they are not sleeping well, you need to do something about it. I remember a patient in a care home who told me that he was not sleeping well. When I discussed this with his carers, they told me that he always slept well and that when he was checked on during the night, his eyes were always closed and he seemed peaceful. It transpired that he did lie still with his eyes closed, as there was nothing to look at in the dark, but he was not asleep, and because he was hard of hearing, he did not hear the carers when they looked in on him. He described how he was scared of the night and would lie there praying for the morning to arrive. When we had asked the doctor to prescribe sleeping tablets for him, and arranged for the carers to go up to him and offer reassurance if he was awake, he was able to get some sleep without feeling so scared. There are many reasons why a patient may not be able to sleep well, including the following:

➤ pain or other discomfort, such as itching, sweating or nausea
➤ the patient's state of mind – anxiety, depression, fear, worry, anger, grief, or anticipating a difficult event
➤ nightmares – these may be due to underlying fear, or they can be a side-effect of some medications
➤ environmental factors, such as noise, discomfort, lighting or an uncomfortable bed
➤ medication, such as diuretics (water tablets) that cause a need to go to the toilet. *Note that if a patient is taking steroids, these should always be given before 2 pm, as they can cause insomnia*
➤ stimulants before settling down for the night, such as alcohol, coffee, large numbers of visitors.

In addition to medication, there are many ways in which you can help your patient to get a better night's sleep.

➤ Ask about their sleep. How do they feel that they sleep and what do they feel might be preventing them from having a good night's sleep?

> If possible, solve the problem, or get someone else in to help.
> Establish a relaxing, familiar bedtime routine.
> Check whether the patient's bed is comfortable, and also check environmental factors such as noise and lighting.
> Some patients have a preferred position for relaxing into sleep. Don't allow concerns about pressure relief to get in the way of this.
> If fear is a problem, it can be reduced by measures such as leaving the door open, turning the bed round so that the patient isn't facing a wall, and providing soft lighting and/or soft music.
> Although alcohol is a stimulant, many elderly people in particular find that a nip of their favourite tipple helps them to sleep. My own father-in-law swore by a glass of whisky at night, and if for any reason he didn't have it, he just couldn't sleep.

Remember: Patients who have a life-limiting disease may be afraid of going to sleep, fearing that they may not wake up. You obviously cannot tell them that this definitely won't happen, but you need to allow them to voice their fears, and to offer them reassurance.

NOISY BREATHING (DEATH RATTLE)

This happens when the patient is nearing death and is due to saliva secretions building up in the patient's throat when they become too weak to cough. The noise from this rattle can be quite alarming for others to hear and family and friends in particular can get very distressed. Explanation and reassurance is very important. It helps to explain what is causing the noise and to reassure family and friends that though it does not sound pleasant, the patient will not be aware of any discomfort and that they will 'not drown' in their own secretions.

A change of position often helps considerably, such as turning the patient onto their side if they can tolerate it. If secretions are evident at the back of the throat or in the mouth, gentle suctioning may be appropriate, but more often than not, the act of suctioning causes more distress than comfort. The most effective measure is to use drugs to decrease the amount of secretions. The two drugs most commonly used are hyoscine hydrobromide and glycopyronium. Both these drugs are equally effective but they need to be used as soon as any rattle is suspected. Both can be given as interval subcutaneous injections or via a syringe driver. Glycopyronium can also be given via a percutaneous endoscopic gastrostomy feeding tube (PEG). (This is a tube that goes straight into the patient's stomach via a hole near to their naval and is used for administering food and fluid.) If you know one of your patients is likely to be nearing the end of life, it is always advisable to anticipate the possibility of noisy breathing and to request a prescription for one of the above drugs. Take advice from your palliative care specialist or doctor as to the dose to use.

Remember: When a patient is nearing the end of their life, their body needs less food and fluid. Reducing food and fluids can lessen the excess fluid in the body and greatly relieve rattle. If your patient is receiving fluids via a drip, either subcutaneously or intravenously, or via a feeding tube, you should take professional advice about reducing, or preferably stopping, this fluid intake. It is important to explain the reason for doing this to family and friends and to reassure them that their loved one does not need extra fluid at this time.

PRESSURE SORES

These are a result of tissue damage caused by unrelieved pressure to a part of the body. Pressure sores usually affect the sacral area (lower back and buttocks), but can also occur on other parts of the body, such as the heel, ear, shoulder and hip. Never underestimate the discomfort that can be caused by a pressure sore. I have known patients who have had very serious illnesses, yet whose greatest source of discomfort was a pressure sore. In care homes, pressure relief is taken very seriously. There are charts that can be used to assess skin condition, and many different forms of pressure relief are available, such as mattresses, chair cushions, bootees, etc. I am not going to discuss this subject in detail, but I want to highlight the fact that a painful pressure sore requires painkiller medication just as much as any other pain. Furthermore, in palliative care, of all forms of care that are given, comfort should always be the priority, so don't place the patient in a position that they find uncomfortable, even if it is to relieve pressure. Try to find other ways of reducing the pressure. When a patient is approaching the terminal phase of life, pressure area care should become less of a priority. When someone is dying, it really does not matter whether they are 'turned two-hourly', so long as they are comfortable.

One very easy pressure-relieving technique that can greatly increase the patient's comfort and only requires minimal movement is a 30-degree tilt movement. This requires a number of soft pillows, usually about four or five, and the pillow edges are placed on one side of the patient under the shoulder, waist area and leg. Another pillow is then placed between the patient's legs to avoid rubbing. There should be sufficient pillows under the patient's head to ensure that their head is in line with the rest of their body. This may require some practice – it helps to rehearse the procedure on someone first. The idea is that one side of the patient's body is eased very slightly off the mattress, thus relieving pressure on that shoulder, buttock and leg. After a reasonable amount of time, the pillows can be removed and placed on the other side of the patient. Very often this manoeuvre can be done by just one person.

SWEATING

Normal sweating is part of the body's natural temperature control mechanism. Excessive sweating can be caused by infection, and can be helped by giving the patient regular doses of paracetamol to reduce fever, and using other body-cooling techniques such as an electric fan or tepid sponging. Unfortunately, some patients may experience excessive sweating due to their particular illness – for example, cancer. This is probably due to chemical factors released by the tumour. Furthermore, patients who are being treated with hormone therapy for illnesses such as cancer of the breast or prostate may suffer from hot flushes and/or sweating. Sweating can also be a side-effect of some drugs, such as morphine. Whatever the reason, you can help by adopting cooling measures such as the following:

➤ ensuring that the patient is wearing cool light clothing
➤ ensuring that cotton clothes and bedding are used if possible
➤ changing bedding and clothing regularly
➤ maintaining an appropriate room temperature
➤ tepid sponging
➤ use of an electric fan.

Remember: A sweating patient will lose fluid, so you need to ensure that they replace this by taking plenty of liquids. Sometimes it is possible to relieve the cause of sweating by changing, stopping or adding to the patient's medication, so always discuss this symptom with your palliative care specialist or doctor.

WEAKNESS

This is a very underestimated symptom for most patients who are in the palliative care phase of their illness. Ironically, it is also one of the symptoms that patients complain about most, using phrases like 'I feel constantly weary' and 'It's such an effort to do anything.' Patients with life-limiting illness often suffer from this weak, weary feeling until they die. You can easily tell the difference between this kind of weariness and the kind that is a result of not getting enough sleep by asking the patient how they feel when they wake up from a sleep. If they say that they don't feel refreshed, then the likelihood is that the weariness is part of their illness and there is little in the way of medication that can help.

However, there are some causes of weakness that can be helped or even reversed, such as:

➤ anaemia (a low iron count in the blood)
➤ depression or low mood
➤ infection
➤ side-effects of some drugs.

If the above causes have been excluded, there are ways that you can help. As I have already mentioned, there is often little in the way of medication that can help with this type of weariness, although some medication can be helpful for some people in the short term. The palliative care specialist or doctor will be able to advise on this (*see* Chapter 10).

Remember: No matter what your level of expertise, so long as you care, there is always something that you can do to help to relieve distressing symptoms for your patient. One of the most important things that you can do is to listen. Acknowledge that the symptom which they are describing is real to them, and assure them that you will do everything you can to help.

CHAPTER 16

Difficult questions

Communication is a vast subject in its own right, and there are whole books, and many chapters in palliative care textbooks, dedicated to communication skills in nursing. Of the various skills that are needed in palliative care, none is more important than the ability to communicate effectively. It would be impossible to include in this chapter everything I have learned about communication skills, and I would therefore encourage any carer to read and learn as much about communication as possible. This chapter is based on some of my interactions with carers and patients with whom I have worked, and hopefully gives a flavour of some of the difficulties that can be experienced, and some of the ways of helping these patients.

Good communication:
➤ helps to ensure that everyone knows what is being said and done
➤ helps to increase understanding and reduce uncertainty
➤ helps to create and maintain trust
➤ reduces anxiety
➤ makes people feel valued.

Bad communication:
➤ means that no one knows what is happening
➤ reduces understanding and creates uncertainty
➤ destroys trust
➤ creates anxiety
➤ makes people feel undervalued.

Many carers find certain situations hard to cope with, and there is seldom anything more challenging than trying to answer a 'difficult' question. Carers

often have difficulty knowing whether or not to talk to a patient about their illness, and not knowing how much, or what, they should say. Some of the reasons why carers might find such situations difficult include the following:
➤ lack of confidence in talking about sensitive issues
➤ lack of training and/or support
➤ fear of showing their own emotion
➤ fear of unleashing emotion in the patient
➤ not having enough time to stop and talk
➤ protecting themselves – not wanting to face their own mortality
➤ fear of harming the patient or making things worse
➤ the need to face their own failure.

Most of us will have heard people say things like 'I don't know what to say', 'I don't want to upset her' or 'I don't think he would cope if he knew.' However, no one really knows how a person will react when they receive distressing news or the painful truth – even if we feel that we know that person really well.

Patients with life-limiting illnesses and their families can ask difficult questions, some of which have painful answers, some of which have uncertain answers, and some of which have no answers.

It can be very difficult to know how to answer a 'difficult' question, and a normal human reaction is to try to avoid or change the subject. However, even if the question asked is not easy to answer, it can be very reassuring to the patient to know that their question has been heard and that they have been given a chance to talk about their concerns.

So what should you do and say if one of your patients asks a difficult question? Equally, what should you not do and say?

It is helpful to:
➤ acknowledge that you have heard the question
➤ show the patient that what they have asked is important
➤ if possible, stop what you are doing, sit down and allow some time to talk with the patient. If you really do not have time to stay and talk at that moment, you should acknowledge the importance of what they have asked and suggest that you come back later to talk to them. Give them a time and stick to it. Leaving a question unanswered like this is not ideal, and you risk 'losing the moment' in which to answer it.

It is not helpful to:
➤ ignore the question
➤ pretend that you didn't hear it

➤ rush to answer the question before thinking about what you are going to say
➤ assume that you know what the patient is asking before you have clarified the question
➤ change the subject ('Oh, look at those lovely flowers your friend brought you')
➤ dash off to attend to something else
➤ look shocked
➤ pass the buck ('Jane will be along later – ask her')
➤ give advice ('Well, if I were you I would do this')
➤ give false reassurance ('Of course you're not going to die')
➤ give a flippant answer ('Well, everyone has to die some time').

Sometimes it is very difficult to know what to say, and if you are really stuck for words, don't panic. Take your time – don't be afraid to be silent for a few seconds while you think about how you are going to answer, and if no words come to you, your very presence and perhaps a touch on the patient's hand or shoulder will show them that you care about what they are asking.

Some 'difficult' questions that I have been asked, and some suggestions about how to answer them, are given below.

A really useful tip, when you are asked a difficult question, is to answer it with a question. By doing this, you are giving the patient time to think about what they are asking, and you are giving yourself some breathing space before you answer.

For example:

Checking the reason for the question
PATIENT: 'How long do I have before I die?'
CARER: 'What made you ask me that question just now?'

Finding out what the patient already knows
PATIENT: 'Have I got cancer?'
CARER: 'What have the doctors told you?'

Never assume anything before you have clarified the question. This is a very easy mistake to make if you don't stop to 'read between the lines.' For example:

Conversation with carer, making assumptions
PATIENT'S HUSBAND: 'She's very upset. How much longer do you think she's got to be like this?'

CARER (MAKING ASSUMPTIONS): 'Well, no one knows for sure, but she is deteriorating and the doctor thinks she may die in the next few weeks.'

SHOCKED HUSBAND: 'I only wanted to know how much longer she's got to remain on her side for.'

Conversation with carer, clarifying the question

PATIENT'S HUSBAND: 'She's very upset. How much longer do you think she's got to be like this?'

CARER (CLARIFYING): 'Are you asking me about your wife's illness or is she upset about something else?'

HUSBAND: 'No, I know all about her illness – I just want to know how much longer you want her to stay on her side for, as she's getting uncomfortable.'

Sometimes the difficult question may come in several parts, with the patient or carer asking you several questions that are all linked together. It can be very difficult to know where to start in responding to such a question, without getting bogged down in a long-winded answer consisting of several parts. The best approach is not to try to answer all of the questions that have been posed. For example:

One option is to answer the question you are most comfortable with

PATIENT: 'Why am I not getting any better? My legs are so wobbly and I don't know why I don't enjoy my food any more. Why can't the doctors give me something to help?'

CARER: 'You've asked several questions. Let me take the one that I feel I can answer most easily.'

Another option is to turn the question around and answer it with a follow-up question

CARER: 'You have asked me several questions. Which one is most important to you and why?'

Telling the truth can sometimes be difficult. Sometimes we don't even know what the truth is. Unfortunately, many questions cannot be answered easily, especially the 'what will happen . . .?' questions. It may seem to the patient that you are avoiding the issue when answering questions like this, but if you are uncertain of the answer, you can only try your best to give as honest an answer as possible. For example:

Leave the patient with some hope without lying to them

PATIENT: 'Will I get more pain towards the end?'

CARER: 'Well, we don't know for sure that you will get more pain. A lot of people don't experience any worse pain towards the end, but we will ask the doctor to prescribe some medicine for you just in case you do feel some pain.'

Don't be afraid to say you don't know the answer

PATIENT: 'Do you think this treatment will work?'

CARER: 'I honestly don't know the answer to that, but I am sure the doctor wouldn't have suggested it if he hadn't thought it would help.'

Don't be afraid to admit to how you are feeling – so long as you don't monopolise the conversation. This shows empathy and compassion. For example:

Admit that you find the question difficult

PATIENT: 'I don't think I'll be here for Christmas, and I want you to tell my family so that they don't go buying me lots of presents. I know what they're like. I'd rather that they heard from you, as you have been so kind to me.'

CARER: 'I'm finding it really difficult talking to you about this. I want to be here for you and your family, but I'm not sure that I can talk to them about Christmas in that way. I know they will be upset, and I will be upset, too.'

PATIENT: 'One of my daughters comes to see me often, which I love, but she often brings her partner with her and I don't like him at all. I don't want to upset her by telling her not to bring him. Could you tell him when he comes that I only want to see my daughter, and ask if he could sit and wait for her.'

CARER: 'Oh, that's a difficult situation for you, but I would not feel comfortable telling him this. I'm not sure how we can get around this easily. Let me think about it and see if there is any way we can deal with this.'

One aspect of communication that carers have told me they find difficult to cope with is silence – for example, when they are talking to a patient about a sensitive subject and the patient suddenly becomes silent. A lot of non-verbal communication occurs during a silence, and if a patient suddenly stops talking, it usually means that they are thinking of something – perhaps something painful that is difficult to express in words. Silence can seem to go on for a long time, and carers have said to me that they don't know what to say or do in these circumstances. It is always helpful to allow silence, but if you start to feel uncomfortable, it helps to say something like *'You've been quiet for a while – what are you thinking about?'* The use of touch can be helpful during a silence, as it helps to 'bring the patient back.' Try offering a gentle touch on the patient's hand or shoulder.

Remember:

➤ The more you read and learn about communication skills, the better you will be at handling difficult questions. You will find some useful reading material in the chapter on 'Further reading, useful websites and other resources' (*see* page 155).

➤ The best way of dealing with a difficult question is by showing your interest and giving your time. Be sensitive, tread carefully, and remember that you are not alone in not knowing what to say. It is not so much about what you say as about the way in which you answer.

➤ There is much value in listening to the patient's story even when there is no treatment available, and what matters most is not what you say but the fact that you care.

CASE STUDY ROSE – THAT DIFFICULT QUESTION

Rose was a 67-year-old woman who had been residing in a nursing home for 3 years following a stroke. She had recovered remarkably well from her stroke, but it had left her with impaired mobility. Having very little in the way of family nearby, she decided to move into a nursing home. Rose noticed that her abdomen seemed to be swelling, and after some investigations, she was diagnosed with cancer of the ovary. Rose was one of those people whom you could not fail to like. Prior to her diagnosis, she was the life and soul of nursing-home life, had a wicked sense of humour and was always ready to take part in any activities that were taking place. She changed almost immediately she received her diagnosis – becoming withdrawn, not wanting to join in with any activities, and seldom coming out of her room. At the beginning, she was not particularly ill and the carers could not understand why she had changed so much. Sue was Rose's key worker at the home, and she was very fond of Rose. She sent a referral through, asking me to visit Rose to see whether I could help. One of the first things Sue said to me when I arrived was 'I just don't know what to say to her any more, and I think I blew it the other day.' Sue went on to describe how she had gone into Rose's room the other morning and Rose had asked her if she was dying. Sue said the question took her completely by surprise and she found herself saying 'No, of course not.' Then her mobile phone had rung and she had left the room to answer it. When she went back into Rose's room, Rose changed the subject away from herself. I talked to Sue about ways of opening up the conversation again, and reassured her that although she might have lost 'that moment', there would be other times to talk. I told her about some of the communication skills she could use, and encouraged her to read some background material on communication. I reassured her that when she understood some ways of responding to difficult questions, the next time would almost certainly be easier. The plan was for Sue to make sure that she had time, and that she didn't have her mobile phone switched on. Then I suggested that she should go and sit with Rose and bring up the 'difficult question' by saying something like 'Rose, when I came into your room yesterday, you asked me a question – you asked me if you were dying. You took me by surprise, and I know I didn't answer you very well, and then my phone rang. It must have taken a lot for you to ask me that question, Rose, and I'd really like to talk to you about it. I've got 30 minutes before I need to start the medicines, and I promise you I haven't got my phone on this time.' When I saw Sue the next time, she explained that she had done as I had suggested and that Rose had opened up and talked to her. She had been able to talk about some of her fears, and although Sue had not been able to answer all of her questions about dying, she was able to reassure Rose about a number of things that were worrying her, such as her fears of going back into hospital, and of experiencing pain. Sue felt very relieved that she had been able to have this conversation, and that she had not ruined her relationship with Rose when she was taken by surprise by that difficult question.

CASE STUDY BRIAN – TIME TO LISTEN

Brian was a new patient in a care home. He was transferred there from hospital, where the doctors had told him and his family that there was nothing more they could do and that he only had weeks to live. From talking to his family, the carers learned that Brian had not had a good experience in hospital. The doctors had taken a long time to come up with a diagnosis, then Brian had contracted a hospital infection, and also his notes had been lost after one of his tests, which meant that he had to undergo that test again. Understandably, Brian and his family were left feeling quite angry.

Brian was a very frail man who couldn't do much for himself, and spent most of his time in bed. He could be quite demanding of the carers' time, and they found it quite difficult going into his room, as he always wanted to talk, and it was always about the same thing – how he had been treated in hospital.

The carers found visits to Brian's room very time consuming, and this posed problems with their staffing levels. I visited Brian, and I was also subjected to a lengthy 'lecture' about his hospital experience. I talked to the carers about ways of handling this, such as giving Brian a set time span when they went to see him, and timing his care to fit in with the maximum staffing levels. Despite these tactics, Brian continued to be a very time-consuming patient, but the carers continued to do their very best to give him as much time as they could. They often said to me when I visited 'We don't have to actually say anything when we are in the room – just the odd word now and again to show we are listening.' Brian eventually died quite suddenly, although very peacefully, five weeks after he was admitted to the nursing home. Not surprisingly, his death was met with a feeling of relief among the carers. Many of them expressed feelings of guilt about the fact that they should be so relieved about not having to listen to his hospital story any more.

After Brian's funeral, two of his daughters visited the home to take a 'thank you' card and a box of biscuits for the staff. They thanked the carers for their patience in listening to Brian. They acknowledged how difficult it must have been to hear the same story over and over again, and went on to say 'When Dad left the hospital, he was very angry and all he wanted to do was talk about what had happened. He often said to us that you carers always had the time to listen to him, and this meant so much to him.'

CASE STUDY JIM – COLLUSION

When Jim was admitted to a care home from hospital he was very frail, having been diagnosed with renal (kidney) failure. He became very breathless with even minimal exertion, and was almost completely dependent on the carers for all of his activities. Jim had a large family who had all gathered together and decided that Jim should not be told how poorly he was. They themselves had been told by the hospital that Jim was dying and that he would probably only live for another 2 to 3 weeks. However, the family felt that if Jim knew this he would just give up. The first thing that they mentioned to the care home was the fact that no one should tell Jim how poorly he was, and that they wanted everything to be as 'normal' as possible. Jim's family used a lot of 'jollying' tactics when visiting Jim, assuring him that he was looking better every day, and encouraging him to eat to build up his strength. Jim's carers found this collusion very difficult, especially as Jim was asking them questions about why he wasn't feeling any better and why he felt so tired all the time. The nurses in the home asked me to visit to help them to deal with this, but when they told Jim's family that they had asked a Macmillan nurse to visit, his family insisted on seeing me first to make sure that I did not say anything out of order. The first meeting took place with Jim's family and his key worker at the care home. It was explained to Jim's family that although they might feel it was a kindness not to talk to Jim about how ill he was, the likelihood was that he was worrying because he knew that he wasn't getting any better. He was asking the carers questions about his health, and this was difficult for them as they didn't know how to respond. Discussion took place about the fact that sometimes not knowing is worse than knowing, even if the news is not good. Sometimes it is acceptable to go along with denial so long as it doesn't seem to be causing anxiety, but when the person concerned starts asking questions, as Jim was doing, it becomes obvious that they are anxious and that they need to have their questions answered honestly. The most important consideration is always the distress of the patient and, as was explained to his family, Jim was showing signs of distress. His family asked how they should tell him how ill he was. The response was that they did not have to tell him directly, but just to be aware of his response when they were talking to him. They were encouraged to answer his questions as honestly as possible. Over the next few days, with a lot of support from the carers, Jim's family were able to talk to him 'differently', and they admitted that once they stopped pretending that everything was fine, Jim seemed more relaxed (and they were, too). He even stopped asking the carers questions about why he wasn't getting better, and just seemed to accept the fact that he wasn't. Jim's family were very relieved that they didn't have to tell him how poorly he was. They could see that merely changing their behaviour when they were communicating with him was enough to give Jim the reassurance that he needed.

CHAPTER 17

Spiritual distress and palliative care

In Chapter 13 on pain, I talked about the concept of 'total pain' and the meaning of physical pain, emotional pain, social pain and spiritual pain. In this chapter, I want to touch on the subject of spiritual pain, as during my work in palliative care I have seen how easily spiritual care can be neglected. I haven't cited many quotes in this book, but I feel that this one deserves to be included in the text. Paul Tournier was a Swiss physician and author who was famous for his work in pastoral counselling. He stated that 'Every disease has two diagnoses – a medical one and a spiritual one.'[1]

I have come across many patients over the years, especially the elderly, who suffer from more than just physical symptoms. For example, they may fear what will happen after they die, or have anxieties or regrets about things that they wish they had done or had not done. This is 'spiritual distress.' Sadly, this type of distress is less likely to be acknowledged by carers, and can therefore escalate into feelings of hopelessness and fear for the patient.

Many carers whom I have met believe that spirituality and religion are one and the same thing. However, this is not necessarily true. The essence of spirituality is about knowing our true selves and what makes our thoughts and beliefs unique to us.

The elderly come to us for care, usually in the last years or months of their life. The focus of our care is usually on what is happening now, and it is easy to 'forget' the years of life experience that each elderly person has behind them. We must not forget that people who have lived a long time have both good and bad memories. It would be lovely for them only to remember the good as they start their journey towards the end of life, but sadly this does not always happen, and for some, bad memories can crowd in, causing spiritual unrest.

It is easy to back away from discussing a patient's fears, due to concerns about 'opening up a can of worms' or not being able to deal with what we have been told. However, helping a patient to die with a peaceful and untroubled mind can be just as important as helping them to die without pain and discomfort.

The following are genuine extracts from patients' conversation which I have heard and that show 'spiritual distress':

➤ 'I'm scared of what will happen when I die'
➤ 'I have so much to sort out – it's not the right time to die'
➤ 'Do you believe there is something after death?'
➤ 'I wish I had been a better mother – it's too late now'
➤ 'My wife will never forgive me for leaving her like this'
➤ 'I never smoked or drank – do you think this illness is some kind of punishment for something else I have done?'

It may not be easy for you to address these issues, but just by acknowledging that you have heard what the patient is saying, and that you realise that what they are saying is very important to them, you will help to reduce their distress considerably (*see* Chapter 16). By listening and showing empathy you will help the patient to feel that someone really cares. You can then help to facilitate further help, such as that described in the following case study.

CASE STUDY TOM – SPIRITUAL DISTRESS

Tom was a patient with end-stage heart failure who had been in a care home for about six weeks. He claimed that he had no family, and his next of kin was a friend who visited once or twice a week. Although he was very breathless for much of the time, Tom generally managed to be quite independent. He was quite a private man, and apart from joining the other residents for meals, he spent most of the day in his room either watching television or reading the paper.

The carers noticed that Tom was starting to look more poorly. He was becoming more breathless and less inclined to join the other residents for his meals. The doctor visited and started him on some medication to help his breathing. The carers made sure that Tom had a fan in his room, and offered to help him with activities such as washing and dressing to try to reduce his breathlessness. At first he declined all offers of help, but gradually, as he became more poorly, he started to allow the carers to help him more. It was while the carers were doing more for him that one or two of them noticed that Tom seemed very low in his mood. He seldom spoke, and seemed to spend a lot of his time just staring out of the window. He seldom slept during the day, and the night staff reported that he did not sleep much at night. The carers asked if he had any problems, but he always said that he didn't. The doctor called to review his medication and felt fairly satisfied that Tom was not in discomfort. He offered to prescribe some antidepressants and sleeping tablets, but Tom declined this treatment. Over the next few days, the carers were concerned that he was becoming increasingly withdrawn, and they felt that he was suffering in some way, but he would not admit to any problem.

I was asked to visit Tom. At first he refused to see me, but gentle persuasion by one of the carers resulted in him reluctantly agreeing to see me. On the day of my visit, Tom was lying in his bed. He seemed very wary of me, or of what I was going to do or say. He made very little eye contact during my visit. I started by explaining my role and going through my usual symptom assessment, in the hope that I might pick up something that was treatable. However, it was fairly evident that his physical symptoms were quite well controlled, even though Tom said very little. I then gently started to ask him what he was finding most difficult at the moment, and how he was coping with this. After quite a long silence, Tom suddenly asked me whether I believed in life after death. I gently turned the question back towards him and asked him what his beliefs were. By continuing the conversation in a gentle probing manner, and allowing frequent silences, Tom managed to disclose that he had done something in his life of which he was ashamed. I asked him whether he felt scared of what might happen to him after he died. Almost with a sigh of relief, he said that indeed he was. When I asked whether he wanted to talk about what he had done, he became quite angry, saying that it was not for a nurse's ears. I asked him whether, if he felt he could talk to someone, who that might be, but he said there was no one who could help. I suggested that a chaplain might be able to help, and I explained how helpful patients in the hospice found the chaplain when they needed to talk. At first Tom rejected this suggestion, saying that he wasn't religious, but I explained to him that he didn't need to have any particular belief, and that chaplains specialise in providing spiritual care for people regardless of their faith. I reassured him that confidentiality would be maintained, and asked him to think about it. I also mentioned that, if he wanted, I could arrange for the chaplain to visit him in the home. The next day one of the carers phoned me from the home to say that Tom had asked me to arrange a visit from the chaplain. Fortunately, the chaplain was able to visit Tom within the next two or three days. One week after the chaplain had visited, the nursing home carers phoned to express their relief at how much more contented Tom seemed to be. Although he was deteriorating, he seemed much more relaxed. He had accepted sleeping tablets to help him to sleep, and all of the carers noticed that he generally seemed to be at peace with himself. Tom died a few days later, peacefully in his room with one of the carers beside him. Neither I nor the carers ever knew what Tom had done that he was so ashamed of, or what he had discussed with the chaplain, nor was it necessary for us to know. The only important thing was that he had been able to die peacefully without fear.

Remember: 'Every disease has two diagnoses – a medical one and a spiritual one.' Sometimes the spiritual distress is not easy to 'diagnose', but failure to recognise and treat it will leave the patient in a state of unease and unrest.

REFERENCE

1 Tournier P. *A Doctor's Casebook.* London: SCM Press Ltd; 1954. pp. 11–16.

CHAPTER 18

The dying process

People tend to die as they have lived. In other words, if they have been happy and contented for most of their life, they will probably accept their dying process in much the same way. On the other hand, if they have been of less even temperament, or life has not been kind to them, they may well display signs of unrest as they go through their dying journey.

In palliative care, we are frequently told that everyone is different. For example, no two people will react in the same way to being told their diagnosis, and no two people will react in the same way to their treatment. Equally, no two people will die in the same manner.

So in acknowledging that there is no 'standard' way of dying, how do we best prepare ourselves, the patient and their family?

Carers and family often want to know 'how long the patient has', so that they can call in other members of the family and plan their activities around being there at the end. This is not always easy to predict, and it is important that you explain to the patient's family and carers that although sometimes we do see changes that may alert us to the fact that the end is near, at other times death can be a sudden event with little prior warning. Taking this into consideration, it is helpful to have an understanding of some of the things that happen to a person when they are dying.

Physically, the body starts to shut down. The person no longer wants or needs food and fluids. This can be a very difficult concept for carers to understand, and they may worry that their loved one will die from starvation and dehydration. However, the body does not require any fuel at this time, and this is nature's way of preparing for death. If you think about plants that die back in the winter, we are generally advised not to feed them, and to reduce watering to a minimum. When a person is dying, their sensations and needs change, so that they no longer feel thirst in the way that we do – the type of thirst that makes us want to drink a glass of water. A dying person does not need to swallow fluid, and simply keeping their mouth moist should allay any discomfort. Therefore, so long as you keep the patient's mouth moist by providing frequent mouth care, and using artificial saliva and lip salves, any thirst-related discomfort will be alleviated. It is important that you explain this to the family, as the provision of food and water is such a 'normal' activity, and not giving food or fluid may seem cruel to them. It may help if you show them how to provide mouth care, as this gives them something positive to do at a time when they are probably feeling helpless. During the dying phase, there is no need to move or turn patients unnecessarily, and it is important that you stop or reduce to a minimum anything that causes discomfort. At this stage, pressure area care is of less importance.

As the body continues to shut down, the patient will sleep more and communicate less. Their extremities, such as hands and feet, may feel cold and look blue or mottled. This is a sign that the circulation is shutting down and that the blood is really only being circulated to the vital internal organs. Urinary excretion will decrease as the kidneys stop working efficiently. Breathing will become irregular and may become shallow, with long gaps between each breath. This is sometimes referred to as 'Cheyne-stoking.' Often, the breathing is accompanied by a rattling sound. This happens because the person is too weak to cough to remove their own secretions. This noise can be very distressing for carers and family, but it can often be resolved simply by changing the patient's position, or by using medication that can be prescribed by the doctor. Again, it is very important to explain what is happening to the family, and to reassure them that although it sounds unpleasant, it is very unlikely to be distressing for the patient. Some people are worried that the patient will drown in their own secretions, but this simply does not happen.

Dying people are sometimes afraid of being alone, and can gain tremendous comfort if someone is with them as much as possible. It may be helpful to leave a door open or a light on to reduce the feeling of isolation. Of course some people prefer to be alone, and it is helpful if their wishes are ascertained before they become too poorly to express what they are.

Of the five senses, vision, hearing and touch are the ones affected by the dying process, with hearing and touch being the last two senses to go.

➤ **Vision.** This may decrease slightly, and sometimes a patient may experience 'visions' of people or events from the past. It is important to acknowledge what the patient is experiencing. Denying that the hallucinations are occurring can often be upsetting and frustrating to the dying person.

➤ **Hearing.** This is the last of the five senses to be lost. It is generally recognised that dying people can hear, even when they are in a deeply comatose state. People who have recovered from comas often describe being able to hear during the time they were in the coma. It is therefore important to talk to the dying person, and to explain and encourage their family to do the same. However, care needs to be taken not to say anything that may upset the dying person if it is overheard. It helps to tell the patient when you are in the room and when you are leaving. Encourage family and friends to do the same, and reassure them that it is OK for them to sit silently, and that they don't need to be talking all the time.

➤ **Touch.** Although the dying person's hands, arms, feet and legs may become increasingly cool, the sense of touch is still present. A person who seems to be in a deeply comatose state will be able to feel touch. It is important to touch a dying person gently, explaining who is touching them, and to explain and encourage the family to do the same.

Sometimes a dying person will appear to be hallucinating, or 'reaching out' to something that no one else can see. Sometimes they may shout or call out, even calling out a person's name. Some dying patients may become restless or fidgety. There is no real explanation for this. The main point is that only the person who is dying knows exactly what is happening to them, and they are experiencing a unique journey, to which those of us watching are not party. So long as symptom control is effective, reassurance given to the family is all that is needed.

If you are caring for someone and you observe some or all of the above signs, you will be able to alert the family to the fact that their loved one is nearing the end of their life. It is a good idea to establish whether the family want to be there when their loved one dies, and to explain the following to them, as I describe from my experience.

In the years that I have been nursing, it never fails to amaze me how, where and when people choose to die. I use the word 'choose' as I believe that this is exactly what they do. I believe that a person who is dying from an illness can sometimes 'choose' the time when they die and who will be present with them when it happens. I have seen a family member sit with their dying relative for hours, and then the minute they leave the room to go to the toilet, their loved one chooses that moment to die. I believe that this happens in order to protect a family member from that last moment of distress. I always explain this to families because, if a relative expresses a wish to be with their loved one when he or she dies, and this does not happen, that family member can feel very guilty and upset. However, if it is explained to them beforehand that dying people seem to 'choose' when they die and who will be there, they may be comforted and protected from feelings of guilt if their loved one dies when they are not in the room.

Although we cannot always provide evidence and proof in nursing care, especially with regard to the dying journey, anything that you as a carer can say to provide comfort to a bereaved person, or someone who is soon to be bereaved, has to be a good thing.

Changes/signs that you might see in a person approaching the final days of life

These include the following:
➤ profound weakness
➤ altered physical appearance – they may look 'drawn', and their skin may be pale or even 'bluish' around the mouth, fingers and feet
➤ urinary and/or faecal incontinence – this can be very distressing to a patient who has always been 'clean'
➤ drowsiness and/or reduced cognition
➤ reduced intake of food and fluids
➤ difficulty with swallowing, usually due to profound weakness.

These signs usually develop over days or weeks, although they can be sudden. However, if this type of deterioration occurs in a patient who has otherwise been quite stable, it is advisable to contact the doctor or other specialist in case there is a reversible cause, such as an infection.

Symptoms that may be experienced during the last few days of life (see also Chapter 7)

➤ **Pain.** Some patients may develop a new pain in the last 48 hours of life. Do not assume that a non-communicative, semi-conscious patient cannot perceive pain. If the patient is taking analgesics (painkillers) orally, and becomes unable to swallow, they must be given their medication by some other route – for example, via a syringe driver. *See also* Chapter 13.
➤ **Agitation, restlessness and/or confusion.** Some patients, especially the elderly, suffer from these symptoms as they approach the end of life. Reassurance and gentle explanation are needed for the patient and their family. The use of sedation is often needed.
➤ **Noisy breathing.** This is often more distressing to carers and relatives who can hear the 'rattling' breathing. Reassure the family and carers.

Changing the patient's position can sometimes help to relieve this symptom.

➤ **Urine retention.** Sometimes people who are used to being continent cannot relax their bladder sufficiently, and the bladder can become very full and uncomfortable. It is important to relieve this discomfort as soon as possible by draining off the urine. This is a relatively pain free procedure whereby a catheter (fine tube) is inserted via the urethra (bladder opening) and the urine is allowed to drain freely into a bag. This procedure needs to be carried out by a qualified nurse or doctor.

➤ **Dry/sore mouth.** This is often one of the most distressing symptoms, but it is also generally the easiest to soothe. *See also* Chapter 14.

Communication with the patient

Communication with dying patients is of paramount importance. Even if you feel that they may not understand everything – for example, if they have dementia, or seem to be unconscious – they will be soothed by your voice. Involve the patient in decision making for as long as possible, and answer their questions honestly. As far as possible, allay any concerns that they may have, such as fears about dying alone or suffering from uncontrolled symptoms such as pain.

Communication with the relatives/carers

Relatives are often reluctant to make their own feelings known, due to fear of upsetting or disturbing the 'busy' professionals. It is easy for nurses and doctors to 'avoid' relatives because they don't know what to say, or they may be worried about upsetting them if they do say anything. However, communication between carers and relatives is important. Even if you do not know what to say, listen to what the relatives have to say. Reassure them that you are doing everything possible to make their loved one comfortable, and that you genuinely acknowledge their distress at this time. Just knowing that you appreciate how they are feeling can be a comfort in itself. Relatives sometimes ask what they can do to help. Offering them something practical to do for their loved one, such as moistening the patient's mouth, can make them feel needed and useful, thus reducing some of their distress.

Being aware of your own feelings

Looking after someone who is dying affects carers differently, and all carers need to be aware of their own feelings about dying, as these can influence the care of the patient and their family. For instance, if you have recently been bereaved yourself, caring for a dying person may bring back painful memories. If you have a close relationship with a particular patient, you might either find that you want to be closely involved in their care, or you might find that difficult. Obviously you can't pick and choose who you can care for at the end of life, but you do need to be aware of your own vulnerability (*see* Chapter 32).

Remember: Everyone is different, and therefore their experience of death will be unique to them. Equally, those looking on will experience what they see and hear differently. You are only responsible for the care that you give, and so long as you feel that you have done your best within your limits of expertise, you probably couldn't have done any more.

CASE STUDY DAVID – A DIFFICULT DYING PROCESS

David was a 63-year-old man with a brain tumour. He was treated initially with radiotherapy and chemotherapy, and was then cared for by his family. Sadly, David was unable to express how he felt, and he started to become aggressive towards his family. When they could no longer cope, he was admitted to hospital. He was then transferred from hospital to a care home after deciding that he didn't want any more treatment. The care home requested my input soon after his admission to support both David and the carers. When he was able to communicate, David frequently expressed feelings of fear and anxiety, especially at night. His gradual deterioration resulted in periods of increased restlessness. He became very unsteady on his feet and suffered frequent falls. He also started to have occasional fits. His needs soon became very complex, as he was having more changes and dose increases in his medication, and was requiring increased levels of nursing input. He was very soothed by the physical presence of another person, but unfortunately his family were not able to visit very often. David started to have difficulty swallowing medication, and there was a danger of him having more frequent fits because he was unable to take his anti-epileptic drugs and steroids. Discussion took place about the need for a syringe driver to be set up, and also about where would be the best place for David to be cared for. Some of the nurses were very keen to look after David in the care home, but others were less enthusiastic, and did not feel confident that they could supply the level of care that David needed. Furthermore, syringe drivers had seldom been used in the care home, and many of the nurses were nervous about using one. A large proportion of nurses were from overseas and, based on their culture in their home countries, believed that David should be in a hospital. Sadly, David was no longer able to express his thoughts about where he wanted to be cared for, but his family wanted him to remain in the care home if possible. The decision was taken to set up a syringe driver, and I went in to help the nurses to do this and to give them training. Because the nurses were unfamiliar with the drugs needed and the high dose ranges we would be using, I spent some time explaining the actions of the drugs and how the dose was calculated. Once the syringe driver was up and running, David settled for large parts of the day, but in between he was often observed to be restless and appeared distressed. He needed frequent interval doses of painkillers and sedation, especially at night. His medication via the syringe driver increased almost every day, and I visited or phoned almost daily during this period, to discuss dose changes with the carers and the doctor. David's overall care was taking up a lot of nursing time, as he needed someone with him almost constantly. The care home was struggling to provide carers 24 hours a day, and David was now too poorly for transfer into the hospice to be considered. He continued to be very restless at times, and although the nursing home brought in extra carers to sit with him, they were very distressed as they watched what they perceived to be an uncomfortable dying process. David's medication continued to be increased daily as he still had periods of restlessness, although these periods decreased in frequency as he deteriorated. He eventually died peacefully three months after being admitted to the care home, and 13 days after the syringe driver was commenced. His family were very grateful for his care, and were especially thankful that he had not been moved into the hospital or hospice. Four days after David's death, the care home held a reflective session with myself and their manager. About 20 nurses turned up – trained and untrained, from both day and night shifts – which was a massive representation from the nursing home. All of the carers were keen to express their views about David's care and to learn from both the positive and negative aspects. Although many of them perceived David's dying process as a 'bad' experience, others felt that he was helped to be as comfortable as possible. I gently reminded them that dying is a unique experience and that they had all contributed to caring for David to the best of their ability. I also reassured them that even in a hospice setting, people do not always die in the comfortable peaceful manner that we would all like to see.

CHAPTER 19

A good death

As sure as we are born, we shall all eventually die. Although most individuals choose not to think too much about how and when their death will occur, most people will want to believe that their death, or the death of someone for whom they care, will be peaceful and pain free.

If you think back to the number of deaths you have seen occur in your care home, you will most probably have witnessed deaths that were seen as peaceful, pain free, dignified, with the family present, etc. Equally, you will most probably have witnessed patients who you felt died less peacefully, perhaps alone, or maybe without the right medication to ease their symptoms. However, it is important to remember that, like most things in life, death is a unique experience, and everyone will experience the process of dying in a different way. What you perceive as being a good death, for someone else may not seem so good.

A good death is the ultimate aim of palliative care. Enabling someone for whom you are providing care to have a good death means involving the person who is dying, and their family, in all decision making. This may include decisions about the treatment given and where that person wishes to die. My experience from working within the care-home field is that most people want to remain in the care home until they die, and many are adamant that they do not want to be admitted to hospital. The care home is their 'home', and is the place with which they are familiar and where they know the people who are caring for them. Furthermore, for some elderly people, death is seen as a natural ending to life, and is often even welcomed.

Sometimes people choose their own way of dying – for example, by refusing treatments or medication – which may go against the feelings and standards of the carers involved. When this happens, it is important to remember that you are not responsible for this person's choice, and regardless of what you feel would be best, you must respect that person's wishes. This type of situation can be very hard to deal with, but so long as you have done your very best to care for the patient despite their wishes, you will have played your part in helping them to have the dying experience they have chosen. Of course, in this type of situation, the carer should be constantly reviewing the patient's wishes to check whether they have changed their mind.

Planning in advance, if possible, is the best way of helping your patient and their family to experience a 'good death.' You need to know what their wishes are, and make sure they are documented so that other carers are aware of what is wanted. Achieving a good dying experience may involve some or all of the following:

➤ having family and friends around, or not – some patients do not want a lot of visitors
➤ having symptoms controlled, but not having to take unnecessary medication
➤ maintaining control over what is happening
➤ not being over-sedated, or choosing to have sedation in order to be more sleepy
➤ understanding the kind of things that might happen throughout the dying process
➤ the patient being allowed to die with their spiritual and cultural preferences recognised
➤ having time to say goodbye to the people whom they choose
➤ not being alone at the end, or actually choosing to be alone
➤ not being constantly disturbed for washes, position changes, etc.
➤ not having their life prolonged unnecessarily – being allowed to go when the time is right for them.

A good death experience in the care home leads to feelings of comfort and good memories.

In contrast to the above perceptions of a good death, a 'bad death' may be seen as:

➤ dying in discomfort or while feeling frightened
➤ an unrelieved 'death rattle'
➤ dying alone
➤ care home staff lacking compassion
➤ spiritual and/or cultural wishes not being respected
➤ the family not getting there in time to say goodbye
➤ a sudden terminal event, such as haemorrhage (*see* Chapter 22), or dying suddenly in the lounge or dining area in front of other people.

A bad death experience in the care home leads to feelings of discomfort and guilt, and negative memories.

Remember: Dying is a unique experience. Whatever the final outcome, you are not responsible for the patient, but only for the care that you give them. Furthermore, your perception of the way in which a person dies is very personal to you, and may be perceived very differently by someone else.

The following case study shows how the carers in the situation were distressed by what they felt was a 'bad death experience.' However, for the patient who was dying, she was doing it her way.

CASE STUDY PAULINE – A DYING EXPERIENCE

Pauline was an 85-year-old woman who had been diagnosed with cancer of the oesophagus, and liver secondaries. She had one son who used to visit her very occasionally and who did not really become involved with her medical situation. She was discharged from hospital to a nursing home to spend her last few weeks of life. While she was in hospital it was documented that she was refusing all medication, and she was therefore discharged with no drugs at all. I was asked to visit by the nursing home, as they felt that Pauline was in a lot of discomfort. They said that she was having difficulty swallowing and that she felt nauseated all the time. She was also constipated, and seemed to be in pain whenever she moved. When I visited Pauline, she looked extremely poorly and frail. However, even as I introduced myself and started to explain why I had come to see her, she was telling me not to bother giving her any medication because she was not going to take anything. Despite my discussing with her how medication would help her symptoms, she was adamant that she would take nothing, nor would she discuss her reasons for refusing. As the days went on, Pauline remained alert and very much in control. If she wanted help she would ask for it, but if help was offered, the likelihood was that she would refuse it. She continued to feel nauseated and constipated. She developed thrush in her mouth, and often seemed to be in pain, but she still refused help. The nurses found this situation extremely difficult and distressing. Being caring, compassionate people, they hated to think that someone for whom they were caring was suffering. In fact they were the ones who were probably suffering the most. The nurses, the doctor and myself discussed what medication might be helpful, and made sure that a prescription was written in readiness should Pauline change her mind. Every day the nurses asked her if she would accept some symptom relief, but her answer was always the same – a polite refusal.

I frequently reassured the nurses that this was Pauline's choice, as someone who was able to make an informed decision. So long as they continued to care for her in the ways that she would accept, and offer medication in case she had changed her mind, they were respecting her wishes and could do no more. Pauline remained very much in control up to a few hours before her death. She never did take any medication, but she allowed one of the nurses to sit with her and hold her hand as she died. That nurse was amazed at how peaceful Pauline was when she died.

CHAPTER 20

After death

The period immediately after a patient's death can be a very emotional time for all concerned, including family, friends, other patients and the carers. This is perfectly understandable, and it is not unusual for carers to feel as though they do not quite know how to react or what to say to the family.

All care homes should have policies and procedures with regard to what to do when someone dies, and of course you should follow these guidelines. Within palliative care, most deaths in care homes, especially of the elderly, are preceded by gradual deterioration and are expected. However, there are many ways in which you can help to ease the distress of family and friends, and indeed the distress that may be felt by others who work and live in the care home.

It is important that people are given as much time as they need to say goodbye to their loved one. After someone has died, there should be no rush to remove the body. Some people may choose to spend a short amount of time at the bedside of the deceased person, whereas others will find it hard to leave the room. Many relatives, especially those with close relationships, such as husbands and wives, derive comfort from just sitting beside the deceased. If this is their wish, support them in what they are doing by giving them time and privacy. Make sure that they can be as close to their loved one as they want to be – for example, by lowering the bed and removing the cot sides – and offer them cups of tea and tissues. Tell them that you will leave them alone for 15 minutes and then you will come back. Usually relatives will be able to leave their loved one by the time you return. However, if a relative is really struggling with the idea of leaving the room, you may need to help them. It can be helpful to suggest that you would like to tidy the room a little and make it more comfortable. Some relatives derive comfort from assisting with last offices, such as helping to wash the body. It is fine to allow them to help if this is their wish. You should also reassure the relative that they will be able to see the body of their loved one as often as they want at the funeral parlour.

When the relative does leave, make sure that they have clear instructions about what to do next. Because distressed people may have difficulty retaining verbal information, it is really helpful if you can give them written information on how and where to register the death, and when they can collect the death certificate. Many care homes have such written information available.

The following information will be helpful to someone who is newly bereaved. (These are general guidelines with which I am familiar for England and Wales. If your care home is in any other area, some of the information may differ.)

➤ If the death was expected, the GP should quite quickly be able to issue a certificate stating the cause of death. This is needed before the death can be registered.

➤ When a person dies in their own home or a care home, their death must be registered within five days in the district where the home is located. This is important, as many residents in care homes may have originally lived in another district.

Most registrar offices have an appointment system, so it is advisable to make a phone call before attending. The registrar will need the following information:

➤ the date and place of death

➤ the full name of the person (including their maiden name) and their last address

➤ the person's date and place of birth

➤ the person's occupation and, in the case of a woman who was married or widowed, the full name and occupation of her husband

➤ if the person is still married, the date of birth of their husband or wife.

When I worked in a hospital, a deceased person's property was handed to the relatives in a grey plastic bag. It was always very obvious to onlookers what this bag contained, and often the contents were visible at the top of an overfilled bag. Your care home may have its own guidance on the packing and handing over of the property of deceased patients, and hopefully this will request the relatives to bring in a small suitcase or carryall, as this is a far more sensitive way of packing and handing over property. Remember also to handle the items you are packing carefully, and to take care how you pack them. There can be nothing worse for someone newly bereaved than to put their hand into soiled clothing, or to find an unwashed denture pot or a packet of opened biscuits.

There is always tremendous pressure on beds in care homes, and often a bed will be filled by someone shortly after the previous occupant has died. In an ideal world it would be preferable to allow at least 24 hours before someone else moves into the room, both as a mark of respect and also to allow the bed and/or room to be thoroughly cleaned and aired. Remember that it can be very distressing for a relative to return to the home shortly after the death and to find someone else already occupying the bed and/or room where their loved one died.

As well as caring for the deceased and their loved ones, it is important to remember others who may be affected by a death in the care home. It may well be that you yourself, or a member of staff who was particularly close to the deceased person, are distressed. That member of staff may not necessarily be a nurse – remember that cleaners and other ancillary workers can also become distressed by the death of someone to whom they had become close. It can be very distressing to return to work and find that someone whom you cared for has died. Also bear in mind other residents who may have known or sat near to the person. Even someone whom you don't think may have been aware of the situation, such as a patient with dementia, can be very upset by a death.

While working with care homes, I have found that some homes tend to 'hush up' deaths from other residents. However, residents – even those with dementia – do notice when another resident is missing. There is no right or wrong way to tell other residents, other than to remember that although death may be commonplace in care homes, there are residents who will be affected. It may be practicable and possible to inform everyone together in the lounge, or perhaps residents can be told individually. A lot depends on the size of the care home and how well the deceased was known, and by whom. Some residents may wish to pay their respects in some way, or may even want to attend the funeral.

Some care homes choose to phone round members of their staff to inform them when a patient has died. This may not always be possible or appropriate, but if you think that one of your staff may be affected by a resident's death, think how you might reduce the shock of them finding out – for example, by meeting them at the door when they return to work.

Remember: Palliative care continues after death in the dignity and respect that are accorded to the body, and in the care and support of the bereaved. Also remember that the way in which you treat the deceased and the bereaved will have an impact on the grieving process of the bereaved.

CHAPTER 21

Acute medical events in palliative care

An acute medical event in palliative care is generally something that can be treated, so long as the patient is not imminently dying. Usually the patient develops symptoms over varying periods of time that alert the general carer that something is not quite right. The following problems can occur in patients who have cancer, and it is important that you as a carer are aware of the symptoms so that you can alert a doctor or a trained nurse who can then help to determine what is happening.

HYPERCALCAEMIA

Hypercalcaemia is a condition in which there is a high level of calcium in the blood. It is most likely to occur in cancer patients who have a certain type of cancer, such as:
➤ squamous-cell cancer of the lung
➤ cancer of the breast
➤ multiple myeloma.

Hypercalcaemia is a fairly common complication of cancer, and it can lead to death if it is not treated. Sometimes the patient is too ill to be treated and it is just a matter of treating their symptoms to keep them comfortable until they die. Hypercalcaemia is sometimes viewed as a gentle path to death, with the patient slipping gradually into unconsciousness. As the calcium level rises, kidney function and conscious levels deteriorate, and coma and death ultimately ensue.

If you are caring for a patient who has cancer, especially if it is of the kind listed above, you should look out for the following signs, which may indicate that the patient has hypercalcaemia:

- drowsiness
- mental dullness
- confusion
- nausea and vomiting
- constipation
- dehydration
- large urine output
- thirst
- anorexia
- muscle weakness.

Many of these symptoms are very common in people with cancer, but if you see a patient with two or more of the above symptoms, you should alert a doctor or other specialist. The diagnosis can be made with a simple blood test and, if the condition is treated, recovery from hypercalcaemia can be quite dramatic. Treatment involves a short period as an inpatient, preferably in a hospice, during which an intravenous infusion is usually given with a calcium-blocking drug and plenty of fluid.

SPINAL CORD COMPRESSION

Spinal cord compression is another acute medical emergency that is again generally more likely to occur in cancer patients. It is caused by any compression or distortion of the spinal cord (the cord that runs inside the length of the spine and controls nerve function). If a patient develops spinal cord compression and it is not treated urgently, they can become paralysed below the waist and end up being confined to a wheelchair for the rest of their life.

Spinal cord compression is more common in the patients with the following cancers:

- breast
- lung
- prostate
- lymphoma
- renal cell (kidney)
- multiple myeloma.

If you are caring for a person with any of the above conditions, the following signs may indicate a spinal cord compression:

- the patient complaining of pain, usually in their lower back
- unusual weakness, and loss of strength in the legs

➤ sensations such as numbness, tingling and pins and needles in the arms or legs
➤ unusual loss of control of the bladder or bowels.

Many of these symptoms are quite common, especially in the elderly, but if your patient has cancer, especially of the kind listed above, you need to mention the symptoms urgently to the doctor or other specialist.

If the patient is well enough, treatment will involve urgent admission to hospital where there are facilities to perform a bone scan. If spinal cord compression is diagnosed, the patient will be given radiotherapy to relieve the pressure on the spinal cord. If there could be a delay in receiving hospital treatment, high doses of steroids may be prescribed.

PATHOLOGICAL FRACTURE

Bone metastases (cancer secondaries) are a common feature of cancer, and can easily result in a fracture, especially following a fall. Bone fracture may also be due to osteoporosis (thinning of the bones), which is a common condition in the elderly. If you see someone fall in the care home, it is likely that they will be checked for signs of injury, including fractures. The patient may even be sent to hospital for an X-ray. However, I want to discuss the type of fracture that can occur in the absence of a fall or injury, which is known as a *pathological fracture*. If a bone is affected by osteoporosis or cancer, it becomes very weak and can easily fracture without the patient having suffered any obvious trauma. Sometimes it can literally happen overnight after turning in bed, or a bone may just fracture on weight bearing. This type of fracture can present with a variety of symptoms, including pain, reduced mobility or acute confusion.

Again, the elderly are very prone to all of these symptoms, but if you are caring for a patient with known disease in their bones, and they develop unusual symptoms as described above, they need to be reviewed by the doctor or a specialist. Unlike the other two acute events, pathological fracture is not a medical emergency, but for the comfort of the patient it is important that they are examined and treated as soon as possible.

Depending on the frailty of the patient, treatment may involve surgery, radiotherapy, or merely symptom control to keep them comfortable.

Remember: If you are unsure whether a patient for whom you are caring has one of the above conditions, always ask for help. Prompt professional attention can make all the difference to the effectiveness of any subsequent treatment.

CHAPTER 22

Acute terminal events in palliative care

Although it is important to include this chapter, I want to emphasise that acute terminal events are not a common occurrence in the care home environment. However, they can happen, so it is important that you understand what is going on and how you can help.

An acute terminal event is the sudden onset of an event that can lead to the patient's death, and will almost certainly cause distress to those observing it. Sometimes such an event can be anticipated and therefore plans can be put in place. However, events such as these can also happen without warning. Distressing acute terminal events such as massive haemorrhage or airway obstruction are rare, and the main aim of your support is to reduce fear in all present, and to reduce the patient's level of awareness. As most such events cause death within minutes, the most important aspect of care is for someone to remain with the patient.

The management and support of most distressing acute terminal events is similar irrespective of the type of event or the cause.

HAEMORRHAGE

Haemorrhage (severe bleeding) is a very rare event, even in hospices. However, sometimes patients who have diseases that may predispose them to haemorrhage are cared for in care homes. Haemorrhage is usually due to erosion of a blood vessel by a tumour.

Patients who may be at risk generally fall within the disease categories listed below:

➤ head and neck cancers, where the tumour may lie close to a major blood vessel
➤ cancer of the bronchus (part of the lung)

➤ gastrointestinal cancer.

Severe haemorrhage is usually a terminal event. Because of the large volume of blood loss, the patient quickly goes into shock, their system shuts down and they usually die very quickly. Because it does happen so quickly, it is highly unlikely that the patient experiences any pain or discomfort. However, for people watching, it can be very traumatic. If you are caring for a patient with any of the above conditions, it is a good idea to get together with the rest of your team and/or a palliative care specialist and formulate a plan to have in place should such an event occur.

In anticipation of the possibility of major hemorrhage, it is certainly helpful to prepare other carers in your team. Sometimes it is appropriate to prepare family members as well. If you are unsure whether they should be informed, seek advice from other specialists such as the palliative care team.

If major haemorrhage is anticipated, it is a good idea to discuss with the doctor or other specialist whether some drugs should be available. These are usually diamorphine (a painkiller) and midazolam (an anxiolytic), which together can help to reduce pain, fear and awareness. However, often the patient dies so quickly that there is no time to give the injection.

One of the simplest things you can do to help to reduce fear and awareness of everyone who is present is to have a red or dark-coloured towel or blanket near the patient at all times. Blood against a white or pale background can look very alarming, but against a dark background it appears less obvious and therefore less shocking to onlookers.

The most important thing to do is to remain with the patient. Do not leave them to go for help. At this time you will be the most valuable and needed person.

Remember: Although major haemorrhage is very rare, it very commonly causes fear among professionals and other carers. Seeing a major bleed can cause emotional distress to those close by, and everyone should be given the chance to discuss the event afterwards.

AIRWAY OBSTRUCTION

An acute airway obstruction is a blockage of the upper airway, which can occur in the trachea (the tube that connects the voice box to the lungs), larynx (voice box) or pharynx (throat) areas. In the palliative care patient, the most likely cause is a tumour compressing the airway. Complete obstruction will rapidly lead to suffocation and death. Although, like a massive bleed, it sounds as if it would be a very distressing event, the patient will quickly become unconscious due to lack of oxygen, and death may rapidly follow. The management and support of the patient and all who are observing are the same as for major haemorrhage, apart from the fact that you will not need dark towels or blankets. Again, the most important thing you can do is to remain with the patient.

Remember: If you are the only professional person present during an acute terminal event, do not leave the patient to get help or drugs. Summon help by pressing a bell, shouting for help or sending someone else to get help. Although the event will be distressing for you, your presence is vital to provide reassurance and care for the patient and anyone else who is present.

CHAPTER 23

Morphine and pain patches

Although this book is not intended to give guidance on drugs and drug doses, I feel that it is important to include a section on morphine and pain patches, as these two methods of pain relief are frequently used in care homes.

MORPHINE

Not unlike the terms 'hospice' and 'Macmillan nurse', the word 'morphine' often alarms people. Morphine is very strongly associated in people's minds with severe pain and death.

Morphine belongs to a group of drugs called narcotic pain relievers, and it is one of the oldest drugs in existence. It is a natural compound obtained from the opium poppy, and is a very effective medication for treating pain.[1]

Morphine comes in different formulations, including capsules, soluble powder, syrup, tablets and injections. Oral morphine is available in two formulations – short-acting and long-acting (sustained-release). Morphine as a short-acting formula is usually prescribed to be taken when needed for breakthrough symptoms, and its effect usually lasts for between 2 and 4 hours. Morphine as a long-acting formula is generally prescribed to be taken twice daily at 12-hourly intervals.

Any patient who is prescribed sustained-release (long-acting) morphine should always be prescribed a short-acting morphine as well to use for breakthrough symptoms.

Diamorphine is a derivative of morphine that is formulated in a white powder form that is diluted and used for injection.

Morphine and diamorphine are usually used to relieve pain, but in smaller doses they can also be used to control the symptoms of breathlessness.

There is no upper dose limit for the use of morphine. Everyone is different, and while one person may need very little morphine to control their symptoms, another person may need a much larger dose.

It is important to remember that morphine does not control all pain. For example, bone pain and neuropathic (nerve) pain may not respond, or only partially respond, to morphine. In these situations other medication may be needed, either in addition to or instead of morphine.

Below are some of the questions that I have been asked by carers when I have discussed using morphine for a patient.

If morphine is prescribed, does this mean that the patient is dying?

Not necessarily. It is not the stage of an illness, but the symptoms that dictate which medicine should be used. We always try to use the least strong medicine first, and then work up to the stronger ones if symptoms remain a problem. Morphine is only used when it is appropriate, and can be used at any stage throughout a patient's illness if their symptoms respond favourably to it. Some patients never need morphine, while others will require it for quite a while. Some patients may need it for a short time to control a symptom, and then when that symptom disappears, they can stop taking it.

Some of our residents still like to drive. Can they still do this if they are taking morphine?

The fact that they are taking morphine does not automatically exclude a patient from driving, so long as their general alertness and concentration are not impaired. It is advisable for the patient to discuss this with their doctor.

Many of our elderly residents enjoy a nip (or more) of alcohol. Will it harm them if they are taking morphine?

No, having a drink of alcohol is not harmful. For many people, alcohol is an enjoyable and normal part of their life. Many elderly people enjoy a tot of whisky or brandy to help them to sleep, and if they are used to this, it is far better than using sleeping tablets. Although it does state on the morphine advice leaflet that alcohol should be avoided, there is no harm in having just a glass or two of what they fancy. The combination of morphine and alcohol may enhance the effect of the alcohol, but so long as common sense is used, there is no need to prevent a patient from enjoying a drink.

Will the patient become addicted to morphine?

No. So long as morphine is used to control symptoms of pain and/or breathlessness, addiction will not occur. Addiction only occurs when people use morphine for recreational pleasure. When used in this way, and in the absence of symptoms, morphine only affects the brain. This is what gives some people the 'high' that can lead to drug addiction.

Should morphine only be used if the pain is severe?

No, morphine should be used as soon as it is needed. Patients should not have to wait until their pain is severe before they are prescribed morphine. It takes longer to work when taken like this, and the patient has to suffer while they are waiting for the analgesic to take effect. The best way to take morphine is 'by the clock', regularly throughout the day, so that a constant level is maintained in the bloodstream to help to prevent symptoms building up. Some people remain symptom free on a stable dose for a long time, while others may need to have their dose increased fairly quickly.

Does morphine hasten death?

No. In palliative care, drugs are not given in doses that will hasten death, but only in doses that will provide symptom relief. However, sometimes when a patient is very ill and nearing the end of life, the administration of morphine can seem to make them very sleepy and they die quite soon afterwards. What is in fact happening is that the morphine relieves the pain and allows the patient to relax enough to let nature take its course. If you think of a time when you have woken in the night with pain, such as toothache, it is impossible to get back to sleep while the pain is present. However, once you have taken a painkiller and it has 'kicked in', your body will relax and you will be able to go back to sleep.

Will morphine cause sleepiness?

Not necessarily. Many people, especially carers, worry that morphine will 'knock the patient out' so that they won't be able to communicate. However, so long as the correct dose is given to control their symptoms, the patient should not become over-sleepy just because of the morphine. Some people do feel drowsy for a few days, but sometimes this comes almost as a relief, allowing the body to get some rest now that the pain is under control. The drowsiness usually wears off after several days.

Does morphine repress the patient's breathing?

No. So long as the correct dose is given to control the symptoms, this does not happen. Indeed, morphine is used to help with breathlessness, and it actually makes the patient's breathing more comfortable.

What side-effects can patients experience with morphine?

Like all medications, morphine does have side-effects. However, there is seldom any side-effect that remains for long, or that cannot be controlled, that would prevent the drug from being taken safely and effectively.

➤ Nausea, if experienced, is usually self-limiting and eases off after a few days. If nausea is likely to be a problem, prescribing an anti-emetic (anti-sickness drug) alongside the morphine for the first few days will nearly always resolve any problems.

➤ Drowsiness will usually subside on its own within a few days as the patient gets used to the morphine.

➤ A dry mouth can be a problem for some patients. Helpful practical measures should be implemented, such as taking sips of water, or using sweets, chewing gum or artificial saliva.

➤ Confusion is very seldom a problem so long as the morphine is given at the right dose. However, elderly patients are less able to tolerate drugs than younger people, due to the decline in kidney function that accompanies ageing. If confusion develops immediately after starting morphine, like the effects of drowsiness and nausea, it should subside after a few days. However, if it continues or is particularly problematic, morphine is probably not an appropriate drug to use for that patient. If confusion occurs when the morphine dose is established, it is unlikely to be due to the morphine, and may be due to an infection or some other cause.

➤ Constipation is the only side-effect that is not self-limiting, and will most probably escalate as and when the morphine dose is increased. Any patient who is started on morphine should *always* be prescribed a laxative, and their bowel habits should be monitored.

ANALGESIC (PAIN) PATCHES

Analgesic patches have a very important role in palliative care, and are widely used and effective for controlling pain. They are very easy to apply, unobtrusive, and the patient can shower and bathe normally while wearing such a patch. There are many different types of patches available nowadays, and the drug involved, dosage, method of delivery and frequency of application differ for each type. The two things they all have in common are that they are absorbed through the skin, and they have a sustained-release action. Because there are so many different patches available in different formats, I do not wish to confuse the reader by naming and describing them all. However, it is important for trained nurses in particular to familiarise themselves with each type of patch that is prescribed. It is also important to remember that once a pain patch has been applied, it will not be effective immediately, as it takes several hours for the drug to build up in the system. Equally, once the patch has been removed, the drug can remain in the patient's body for several hours.

Remember:
➤ The right dose of morphine is the dose that controls the patient's symptoms.
➤ Morphine is safe and effective when prescribed properly and in the right dose.
➤ Morphine does not hasten death.
➤ When starting a patient on morphine, a laxative should *always* be prescribed at the same time.
➤ When pain patches are used, it will take several hours after the initial application before the drug starts to become effective, and once the patch has been removed, the drug can remain in the patient's body for several hours.

REFERENCE

1 science.education.nih.gov/supplements/nih2/addiction/other/glossary/glossary2. htmhttp://www.drugs.com/morphine.html (accessed 11/1/2008)

CHAPTER 24

Dementia

This chapter describes the difficulties that can arise either for a patient who already has dementia and is then diagnosed with a life-limiting physical illness, or for the patient who develops dementia as a result of their life-limiting illness, as may for example occur as a result of a brain tumour or a stroke. Many patients in care homes are affected by dementia, which means that caring for these people can sometimes be very challenging. For many people, the elderly in particular, dementia is a life-limiting illness, but the trajectory of the illness is often quite long – extending over months, or even years. This means that the patient affected may have uncomfortable symptoms for a long time. However, these patients are less likely to receive palliative care support than are those who are suffering from other life-limiting illnesses.

Dementia is defined by the World Health Organization (WHO) as:

> A syndrome caused by brain disease, usually of a chronic or progressive nature, in which there is a disturbance of multiple higher cortical functions, including memory, thinking, orientation, comprehension, calculation, learning capacity, language and judgement. Consciousness is not clouded. The impairments of cognitive function are commonly accompanied, and occasionally preceded, by deterioration in emotional control, social behaviour, or motivation. This syndrome occurs in Alzheimer's disease, in cerebrovascular disease, and in other conditions primarily or secondarily affecting the brain.[1]

Overall, dementia is a general term used to describe different types of diseases that affect the brain. Dementia damages the brain over a period of time, causing a progressive loss of brain tissue, which cannot be replaced. Each person will respond differently to their illness, depending on which area of the brain is damaged. For example, the frontal lobes at the front of the brain are what are considered to be the emotional control centre. An individual who has damage to the frontal lobe may therefore display significant personality changes.

Many patients in care homes are affected by varying degrees of dementia, and this can affect their ability to describe how they are feeling, due to factors such as:

➤ memory loss, especially short-term memory
➤ inability to concentrate
➤ difficulty in finding the right words or understanding what other people are saying
➤ disorientation in time and place
➤ mood changes and behavioural changes.

Carers will be only too aware of the differing behaviours displayed by patients who have dementia, such as those who wander around a lot, or those who show repetitive behaviour. Very often carers come to understand what the various behaviours mean, and can work out what the person wants and respond to their needs accordingly. However, for a patient with dementia who is diagnosed with an illness such as cancer, it can be very difficult to distinguish between their 'normal behaviour' and any behaviour which may indicate that they are in distress. If a patient with dementia for whom you are caring shows unexplained changes in behaviour and/or signs of distress, you should consider whether they might be in pain, or suffering from another symptom, such as nausea, constipation, itchy skin or some other discomfort. The use of a pain/distress assessment tool can be very helpful, and it also helps to keep a record of what the patient may be feeling, even if they cannot express this verbally, and what kind of therapies may be helpful. There are various pain/distress assessment tools available, some of which can be downloaded from the Internet. Some are given out by pharmaceutical representatives and relate to the product that they sell. One of the assessment tools that I find very useful for patients with dementia is the Abbey Pain Tool. This can be used to measure pain in people with dementia who cannot verbalise, and can be used both as an assessment tool before intervention, and to measure the effectiveness of the therapy given after intervention (*see* Chapter 13).

The important points to remember when using a pain/distress assessment tool can be summarised as follows:

➤ The tool is only as accurate as the people who fill it in.
➤ Because everyone is different, what might work for one person might not work for another.

Sometimes it is much better to make up your own distress assessment tool based on the person as you know them (*see* Figure 24.1).

Name:	Elsie White			
Date	**Time**	**Medication**	**Behaviour**	**Carer's action**
1/1/08	9 am	Paracetamol 2	Sitting quietly	No action needed
	11 am		Fidgeting with her clothes	Taken to toilet. Passed urine and a little wind
	1 pm	Paracetamol 2	Sleepy	Helped with her lunch. Ate a little of her mash and veg and her pudding
	3 pm		Family visiting. They came to say they think she is in pain as she is restless	Explained that it is not time for her next dose of paracetamol, but that she could have some morphine
	3.15 pm	Oramorph 5 ml		
	4 pm		Family came to say they are going now as Elsie is asleep	Elsie asleep. Looks comfortable

FIGURE 24.1 Elsie's chart.

When providing palliative care for a patient with dementia, it is important to try to be prepared. Find out what kind of symptoms might occur and what you should be looking out for – for example, signs of distress that may indicate constipation as a result of taking painkillers. If you are uncertain whether or not your patient is displaying signs of distress, always ask for a doctor's assessment or input from the specialist palliative care service.

Remember: If a patient without dementia experiences discomfort from an illness, then you should assume that a patient with dementia will feel discomfort too.

CASE STUDY ELSIE – PAIN IN DEMENTIA

Elsie was an 84-year-old woman who lived in a residential care home. She was diagnosed with vascular dementia two years prior to her admission to the home, and had been looked after by her husband. When he died, her family helped her to move into a residential home nearby. For the first nine months, Elsie was fairly settled. Although she didn't talk, with help from her family her carers came to understand what her various behaviours meant. For example, if it became too noisy for her in the lounge area, Elsie would put her hands over her ears and rock backward and forward in her chair. This was the cue for the carers to take her back to her room for some peace and quiet, where she would relax. If Elsie started to wander, the carers knew that she needed something, such as a drink, or the toilet, or that she was too hot or cold, and they could attend to whatever her need was.

Elsie developed a chest infection that was treated with antibiotics, but she didn't seem to get any better. She was admitted to hospital, where tests showed that she had a tumour on her lung. In view of this and the results of blood tests, the doctors felt that she almost certainly had cancer. However, it was decided not to proceed with any further investigations or treatment due to Elsie's frailty, and she returned to the home. I was called in shortly after she had returned because the carers had noticed changes in her behaviour. Elsie still got up to wander around, but now she seemed agitated, and the carers found it difficult to identify what she wanted. In addition, she wasn't sleeping so well at night. She was unable to communicate verbally what the problem was, and she would not sit or lie down for long enough to allow either myself or the doctor to examine her. I established from her carers that her bowels were functioning normally and that she was passing urine easily. She didn't seem to have an infection, so I had to assume that she was uncomfortable in some way. The doctor prescribed some painkiller medication for her, and after two days the difference was quite dramatic. Elsie was no longer agitated and seemed quite content to sit in her chair or lie on her bed.

I discussed the use of a pain/distress assessment chart with her carers, and also advised them about other possible signs and symptoms to look out for, such as breathlessness and constipation. Some of the carers got together and designed a very simple but effective chart (*see* Figure 24.1) that they filled in to record Elsie's behaviours in relation to the medication that she was taking. From this it soon became apparent that she needed to take a stronger painkiller. One night, Elsie kept opening the cupboard door next to her bed. This behaviour continued for several nights, and she became more and more agitated every time someone closed the cupboard door. One of the carers noticed that she seemed breathless, and remembering the discussion about signs which might mean that Elsie was feeling distressed, she put an electric fan in Elsie's room. It turned out that she was thinking along the right lines – Elsie was indeed becoming breathless, and it may have been that she was opening the cupboard door because she thought that it was a window. She seemed to find the fan soothing. Over the next few weeks, Elsie gradually became weaker and started to spend more time in bed. She was sleeping more and eating less. She was now on a pain patch and taking oral morphine very occasionally, mainly before the nurses washed and changed her. The district nurses started to visit her and helped out by providing pressure-relieving aids. One evening, Elsie's family were sitting quietly by her bed when they noticed her breathing change. Within minutes, as they sat with her, Elsie simply slipped away very peacefully.

CASE STUDY BILL – DIFFICULTY USING A PAIN/ DISTRESS ASSESSMENT TOOL

Bill was a 69-year-old man who was living a happy, healthy life until he was diagnosed with a brain tumour. Despite treatment, because of the type of tumour he had and the area of the brain that it was affecting, Bill developed dementia. Sadly, the dementia was so severe that Bill's family simply could not manage his care at home, and he was admitted to a nursing home. His dementia manifested mainly as obsessive-compulsive behaviour and periods of acute agitation. Outwardly, he appeared quite fit and healthy, being strong in stature and having a healthy appetite, but inwardly, his dementia was progressing until it reached the stage where Bill could no longer associate an object with its purpose. For example, he knew when he needed the toilet, but he could not associate the toilet with his need to urinate, which meant that he sometimes urinated in the sink or other receptacles. Bill knew that he wanted to eat, but the knife and fork on his tray became meaningless to him, and he would try to cut his food with paper tissues, or a newspaper. His family and carers watched sadly as his illness progressed and day-to-day items of living became increasingly less familiar to him. It was difficult to know when Bill was in pain or other discomfort and, if so, where he was feeling it, as he would become agitated and say things like 'I've got pain in my toothbrush' or 'this shoe is stinging.' In contrast to Elsie's case described above, the use of a pain/discomfort assessment chart for Bill was of no help, as he seldom used the same words or actions to interpret what he was feeling. The care staff decided to try to restrict the number of people helping with Bill's care to only two or three familiar carers, so that he was not having to deal with a lot of different faces. They tried to keep a set routine for him, so that meals were always served at the same time, and getting up and going to bed happened at a set time. Bill was given regular painkillers rather than having to wait while someone tried to assess whether or not he was in pain. By keeping to this routine as much as possible, Bill's care was managed as best it could be. It was often a fine line between not wanting to over-sedate him and wanting to ease his mental discomfort. Over a period of approximately three months, Bill deteriorated to the point where he could do very little for himself and needed one-to-one nursing care. He was given medication via a syringe driver, and eventually died peacefully with his family present.

Although Bill's particular type of dementia created many nursing challenges, by making a very individualised palliative care plan for him, he was enabled to remain in the nursing home until he died.

CASE STUDY MAISIE – USING DISTRESS ASSESSMENT CHART AND OBSERVATION TO HELP THE DOCTOR

Maisie was a 97-year-old woman with severe dementia. She was bed bound, doubly incontinent and unable to communicate verbally. Normally quite an 'easy' patient to care for, it was a surprise to everyone when she suddenly started to squeal very loudly. This squealing could go on for periods ranging from a few seconds to minutes at a time, and was worse after any disturbance such as washing and changing. The carers asked for a visit from the doctor, but he didn't feel there was a problem and was reluctant to prescribe any medication. The other residents, especially those who occupied nearby rooms, started to complain about the noise. It was at this point that I was asked to visit to assess Maisie. However, throughout my visit she was actually very quiet and relaxed. While she was so relaxed, I asked one of her carers to record her pulse and blood pressure, both of which were found to be within the normal range. We discussed any other changes that they observed when Maisie was squealing, and one or two of the carers said that she seemed to frown quite a lot. I asked the carers to draw a chart on which they could describe facial expressions, and I suggested that they should fill this in both when Maisie was relaxed and when she was restless, so that we could try to assess what the problem was. I also asked the carers to continue to monitor her pulse when she was agitated. The next day, they phoned me to say that they had recorded these observations three times when Maisie was squealing, and each time her pulse was fast and she seemed to be frowning. Armed with this information, I discussed the observations with the doctor and suggested that we should try Maisie with a small-dose pain patch (as she was very reluctant to swallow medicine). After 24 hours on this analgesia, Maisie appeared very much better. After a further two increases in the dose of the pain patch, she stopped squealing. She became much calmer generally, and even started to eat more.

REFERENCE

1 World Health Organization. *International Classification of Diseases. Version 10.* Geneva: World Health Organization; 1994.

CHAPTER 25

Palliative care for people with learning disabilities

The provision of specialist palliative care for patients who are affected by varying degrees of learning disability is generally increasing. The improved life expectancy of people with a learning disability means that they are more likely to develop a life-limiting illness at some stage of their life. Sadly, people with learning disabilities often end up in hospital for end-of-life care because their carers lack knowledge of palliative care and feel unsupported. However, by working as a team across the professions, it is perfectly possible to enable carers to provide care for such patients in their home environment.

Whilst helping to support patients with learning disabilities, I have learned from their carers the importance of being aware of that patient's particular way of communication and the different ways that they may express discomfort. For example, one young man I helped care for often shouted out, squealed and grunted. This was 'normal' behaviour for him. However, if he was in discomfort, he displayed this by being quiet and poking his tongue out of the side of his mouth. To me, this quieter behaviour was more normal than when he was shouting and grunting. I was very grateful that his carers were able to interpret his behaviours so that together we could eliminate his discomfort. On another occasion I was introduced to a young lady with learning disability and profound physical disability. On touching her hand, she grimaced and 'squealed out.' I was alarmed, thinking that I had hurt her. However, her carer told me that this was her way of expressing pleasure.

Like patients with dementia, people with learning disabilities have varying levels of comprehension and ways of expressing themselves, and often the people who understand them best are their carers.

Some of the behaviours that are used by people with learning disabilities to express themselves include the following:

➤ vocal responses and sounds, such as crying, moaning, squealing or grunting
➤ physical responses, such as rocking, pacing or hand gestures
➤ facial expressions, such as grimacing
➤ withdrawal and/or low mood
➤ disturbed sleep patterns
➤ self-harm, such as head banging
➤ hyperactive behaviour.

Often the above behaviours will be displayed for positive reasons, such as the squealing and grimacing I described above. However, when looking after a person with learning disabilities who also has a life-limiting illness, it is very important to be able to interpret the meaning of any changes from their normal behaviour in case these are an indication of pain or other distress. Using an 'observe and react' technique by people who know the patient best is one of the best ways of interpreting and treating symptoms in these patients.

The carers with whom I have worked have found the use of pain/distress assessment tools very helpful when trying to identify signs of pain and distress. Sometimes, well-researched tools such as those I have included in the chapter on 'Further reading, useful websites and other resources' (*see* page 155) will prove more than adequate. However, whichever tool or chart is used, it should meet the needs of the person affected and of those who are caring for that person.

Remember: Providing palliative care should always involve a high standard of communication and teamwork, but especially for a patient who has learning disabilities, it is important that the carers' expertise and input are valued, and that all of the professionals involved work together. The following case studies concern real-life situations that highlight the importance of working together, and the use of a personalised tool for assessing distress.

CASE STUDY MICHAEL – THE IMPORTANCE OF WORKING TOGETHER

Michael was a 54-year-old man who lived in a care home for people with learning disabilities. He had been cared for in various institutions for 40 years, but was now very settled in his current home, which he shared with ten other people and their carers. After he had been generally unwell for some time, Michael was diagnosed with a rare cancer that affected his colon (the lower part of the digestive system). He had severe learning disability, with high levels of anxiety and challenging behaviours. His peers in the care home also suffered from severe disability and complex behaviours. Understandably, Michael's carers had very limited knowledge of palliative care, and they did not know how to explain what was happening to Michael or his peers. Michael's mother was the only relative in contact with him, and she had her own mental health issues. However, she was adamant that Michael was cared for in 'his home' if at all possible. Typical of many people with severe learning disabilities, Michael only really felt secure if there were people around him whom he knew. Strangers upset him and hospitals really frightened him, even though the carers were always with him when he went to the hospital. Michael's carers were not at all sure that they would be able to care for Michael, and they were understandably anxious. Michael's doctor suggested that they should contact the Macmillan nurses, and this is when I became involved. Having no experience in caring for people with learning disabilities, I worked closely with Michael's carers, using their communication skills to determine the best type of care for Michael.

The different professions worked together as described below.

Specialists from the learning disabilities sector helped by:
- supporting Michael and developing a programme to look at his own and his peers' understanding of the issues
- attending multi-disciplinary meetings with Michael's carers and advising on issues of concern
- advising the home and other healthcare professionals about consent and capacity issues
- advising the carers and other healthcare professionals about monitoring and recognition of pain in individuals with a learning disability
- supporting Michael's mother
- undertaking bereavement work with Michael's peers after his death.

Specialists from the medical sector, Michael's GP, his consultant, district nurses and Macmillan nurses helped by:
- facilitating communication between the learning disability professionals and the medical professionals
- providing staff support in the form of education and training in the principles of palliative care
- coordinating symptom control for Michael
- training and practical demonstrations on specialist equipment that was needed for Michael, such as pressure-relieving aids and a syringe driver.

Together, the learning disability carers and the primary care team combined their respective expertise and knowledge, while acknowledging each other's skills and limitations. Thus the pressure of caring for someone in a difficult situation was shared. The result was that Michael was able to remain in his home with his peers and carers until his death. His mother was able to gain support from the home, and was present, together with Michael's key worker, when Michael died. His death was perceived as being dignified and peaceful by both his mother and his carers. The loss of Michael and its effect on his peers was recognised, and learning disability bereavement counsellors were called in to support these individuals.

CASE STUDY FRANK – PERSONALISED CARE BOOK

Frank was a 42-year-old man with severe learning difficulties. He lived in a care home with six other people with similar disabilities, supported by carers 24 hours a day. Over a period of a few weeks, Frank's carers noted that he seemed unwell. He was losing weight, he sometimes seemed to be breathless, and he had a cough that was not responding to antibiotics and cough medicine. Following tests organised by his doctor, Frank was found to have lung cancer. A decision was taken jointly by the medical professionals, Frank's next of kin and his carers that it would not be in Frank's best interests to perform further investigations or to give active treatment such as radiotherapy or chemotherapy, as he became very distressed by anything or anyone medical. It was felt that Frank would be best cared for in the surroundings that he knew with the people whom he regarded as 'his family.' Frank's normal routine during the day was quite active. He liked going to the pub for lunch with one of his carers, he loved to visit the cake shop, and at regular intervals throughout the day he enjoyed a cigarette. Frank also had a lady friend who lived in the same home. I was asked to be involved right from the start to help to support the carers who were looking after Frank. Following an initial meeting, it was decided that the best thing the carers could do for Frank was to keep his routine as normal as possible, but to be alert for any changes which might indicate that he was uncomfortable or in distress. The carers discussed the use of a pain/distress assessment tool, and looked at some of the charts. However, they felt that that such a chart might be difficult for the non-nursing carers to interpret, so they decided to talk together and come up with something that would work for all of them. After discussion, they produced 'Frank's Book', and each of them wrote in it as and when they wanted if they had any concerns, or if they felt that something wasn't quite right. Because the carers knew Frank so well, they were the best placed people to observe any changes in him. Frank trusted them, but he had a real fear of medical professionals, myself included, and would become very distressed if a nurse or doctor was near him. He would hit his head quite hard with his hand and keep saying 'I'm all right, there's nothing wrong with me.' I met with Frank's carers and discussed the types of problems that Frank might encounter due to his illness. Because his lungs were affected, it was likely that he might become breathless. Because of the location of the tumour, there was a possibility that he might cough up blood. In general, he might become more tired and go off his food. We talked about the importance of not alarming Frank if they did notice any symptoms, but instead seeking advice from the doctor or myself. At the time of diagnosis, the only medication that Frank was on constantly was an anti-psychotic drug (a drug prescribed to help to reduce distressing behaviour) that he had been taking for years. He was used to this and took it without any problem. However, any other medication alarmed him and made him very uneasy. Therefore, knowing that Frank would almost certainly require medication during his illness, the decision was taken to start him on a small dose of oral morphine liquid regularly, as this would help both his cough and his breathlessness. It was important for the carers not to lie to Frank about why he was having this medicine, so it was decided to tell him that the morphine liquid was to help his cough, which was true. After initial wariness, Frank accepted this and got used to taking the liquid regularly. The carers were surprised how much better he seemed after he had been taking the oral morphine for a few days. One day, one of his carers noticed some blood around Frank's mouth. At first she thought that he might have scratched himself, but having been alerted to the fact that he might cough up blood, she reported what she had observed to the other carers, and wrote it down in 'Frank's Book.' This observation did turn out to be 'haemoptysis' (coughing up blood), and a decision was taken to have some medication and resources nearby for emergency use if Frank did go on to have a major bleed (*see* Chapter 22). The GP prescribed a course of antibiotics for Frank that would help if any infection was present. Frank accepted these without problem. Although the carers were alarmed about the blood, Frank did not seem in the least concerned, and the carers did a wonderful job of keeping their fears from him. Shortly after his course of antibiotics, it was noted that Frank had lost his appetite – especially for the sticky cakes that he usually really enjoyed. His carers were advised to examine his mouth, if he would let them, as he probably had thrush (an oral fungus that is quite common, especially after a course of antibiotics) (*see* Chapter 11).

Frank was quite reluctant to have his mouth inspected, so the decision was taken to prescribe some anti-thrush medication anyway, based on the fact that it would help if he had thrush and would do no harm if he didn't. Frank was becoming quite good at accepting medication, so long as he understood what he was taking it for. He was told that this medicine would help to stop his mouth getting sore. After 10 days, Frank was enjoying his food again. The carers who worked overnight started to report that he was not sleeping as well, and that he would often come out of his room and lie on the sofa in the lounge area, and would be restless. When they asked him whether he had any pain, he would become very agitated, saying 'I'm all right, there's nothing wrong with me.' A meeting was arranged for me to attend to discuss with all of the carers the possible reasons for this particular change in Frank's behaviour. The possibilities were that he was in pain, or that he was finding it difficult to breathe when lying flat, or that he was scared of being alone. The carers who knew him really well felt that he was scared, as even during the day he was trying to remain near to one of them for much of the time. Based on their observations, the decision was taken to increase Frank's morphine dose and to give him a 'sustained-release' formula, using the liquid morphine for instant relief when necessary (*see* Chapter 23). If Frank was experiencing any combination of pain, breathlessness or feeling scared, this increased dose would help. If after a few days he seemed to show no improvement, then we would try something different. However, the increase in the morphine dose did help, and although Frank continued to sleep in the lounge, his sleep was observed to be more restful. Using the 'observe and react' technique by people who knew him was working really well, and all of the carers felt increasingly confident and reassured that they could understand the 'signs' Frank was giving by his changes in behaviour, without the need to ask him endless questions that would cause him unnecessary distress.

CASE STUDY KATY – PERSONALISED PAIN CHART

Katy was a 32-year-old woman living in a care home for people with learning disabilities. While a carer was helping her to bathe one morning, Katy was found to have a lump on her right breast. Katy's parents, who were very involved with her care, decided that she should know what was happening, and they gently discussed and described everything that was happening as Katy underwent various tests, which culminated in her undergoing surgery to remove her breast. Throughout, all explanations were given at Katy's level of understanding, and she coped extremely well, coming through her surgery and returning to good health remarkably soon afterwards. However, during the various tests it was found that Katy's cancer had spread to other organs in her body, and that the type of cancer she had was a particularly aggressive one. This time, Katy's parents took the decision not to tell her about the spread of the disease. The rationale behind their decision was that she seemed remarkably well and had really 'bounced back' after her surgery. They understood that, to Katy, the breast lump was visible and tangible and she could comprehend the fact that she had a cancer there that needed to be removed. However, the fact that the cancer was also in her lungs and her liver was not visible or tangible to her, and therefore while it was not causing her a problem, they felt that she didn't need to know about it. A discussion took place between her parents, her carers and the palliative care team as to what types of signs to be alert for that might indicate Katy was worried, or needed to know more about her illness. The decision was taken that as and when she asked questions, or showed signs that something was bothering her, her parents would be the ones who talked to her. They were very keen that no one should lie to her or give her false reassurances. Katy spent a remarkably happy and apparently healthy six months. She went for her regular check-ups with the cancer specialist and was very proud to tell anyone who asked about 'her doctor and nurse friends' and about her specially made boob! Just after Christmas, about eight months after she had been diagnosed, Katy's behaviour started to change. She had always been quite volatile when she was excited (for example, when her favourite football team was playing), but she was becoming more so for no particular reason. Her carers who slept by her overnight also reported that she seemed quite restless in her sleep. Her mother was the first to identify that Katy seemed to be experiencing pain in her shoulder. Everyone's fear was that the cancer had spread to her bones. However, subsequent scans revealed no sign of this, but the spread of cancer in her lungs was more significant, and it was thought that her pain might be related to this. Everyone who knew Katy was aware that she had a high pain tolerance, seldom complaining of cuts and bumps, and sailing through her breast surgery with very little apparent discomfort. They were worried that the change in her behaviour was an indication that she was in pain. Katy's doctor started her on some painkillers, and the Macmillan nurse suggested the use of a pain/distress assessment chart to show whether this medication was effective. Katy's mother looked at some of the various charts – both well-known researched tools, and others that had been made up for other patients. She felt that Katy was capable of filling in a chart herself, but in order for her to do this, and to continue doing so, it had to be simple and easy to fill in, and interesting enough to 'excite' her. She therefore designed a chart with rows of faces with eyes and a nose but no mouth. All Katy had to do was draw in the mouth expression. Because Katy's operation had been on her left side, but the pain seemed to be in her right side, her mother decided to draw a left and a right side for Katy to fill in (*see* Figure 25.1).

Name: Katie...................................... **Date:** ....

Time	Left	Right
9.00 am	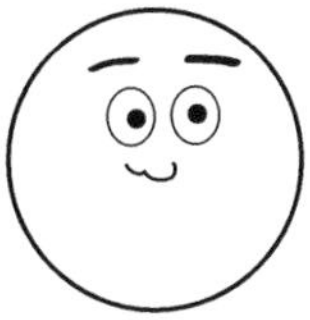	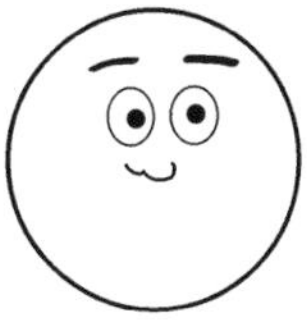
12:00 Midday	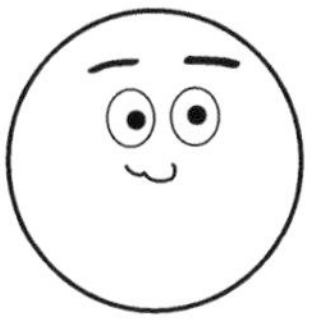	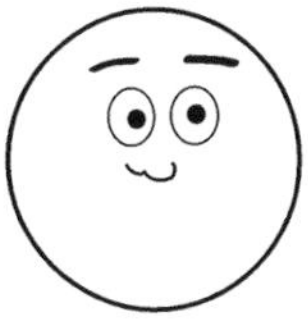
3.00 pm	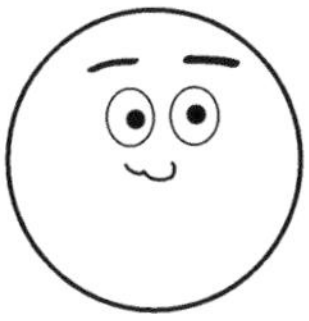	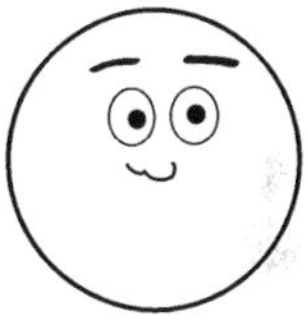
6.00 pm	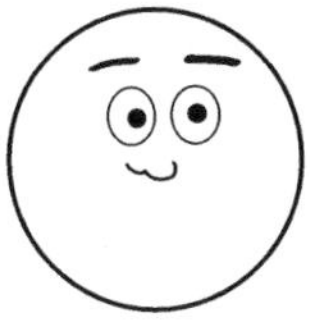	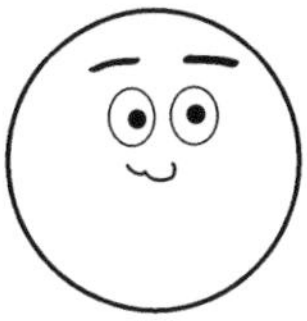
9.00 pm	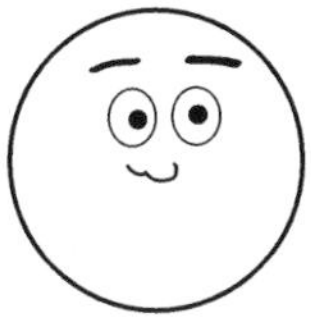	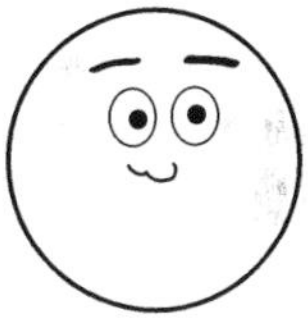

Draw in: A smiley face if it doesn't hurt at all.
A plain face if it only hurts a little.
A sad face if it hurts a lot.

FIGURE 25.1: Katy's chart.

Katy was very enthusiastic about this chart and felt 'very important' to be filling it in. Anyone who went to visit her was shown the chart and given a full explanation of what the faces meant.

Although Katy very seldom verbally complained of pain, this very simple chart clearly showed whether she was experiencing any discomfort. Katy's mother and her carers were able to monitor her reaction to the painkillers and report their observations to the doctor.

CHAPTER 26

The unexpected

Although it would be helpful if we in the medical profession were able to predict disease progression, people and diseases remain very unpredictable, and often surprise us.

Figures 26.1, 26.2 and 26.3 are three well-documented charts that show the general predicted disease trajectory in three main groups of life-limiting illnesses. Figure 26.1 shows how patients with cancer often have quite a high level of function initially, but how once they start to decline, death occurs quite quickly. Figure 26.2 shows how patients with organ failure, usually heart and lung failure, generally have a poor functional status, and their disease path goes up and down, often with periods of inpatient care. Death usually seems to occur quite suddenly. Figure 26.3 shows the elderly frail group of patients, often with dementia. Their level of function is generally much lower than that of the other groups, but their overall trajectory is much more gradual. These charts are used to help medical professionals to 'plan' end-of-life care.[1]

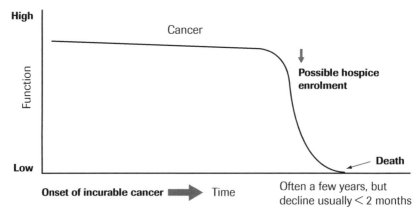

FIGURE 26.1 Cancer trajectory.

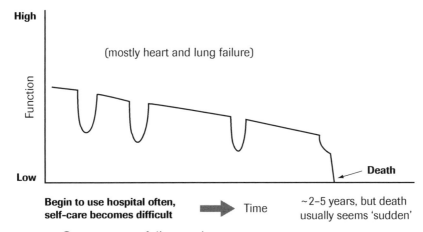

FIGURE 26.2 Organ system failure trajectory.

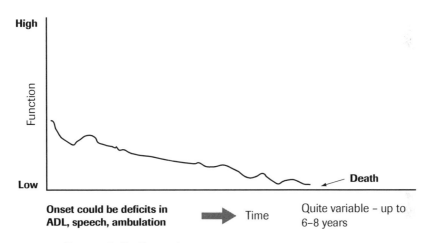

FIGURE 26.3 Dementia/frailty trajectory.

However, by the very nature of their physical and spiritual make-up, each person is unique, and certainly does not live their life according to a chart. Sometimes we see a patient who we feel fairly certain will die quite quickly, and we are surprised when they carry on living beyond expectation. On the other hand, we also see those who we feel have a fairly good prognosis, and they suddenly die. With any life-limiting illness, complications can arise that can have a quite sudden fatal outcome, such as embolism (blood clot) or sudden haemorrhage. However, apart from such life-destroying complications, what never fails to amaze me, even now, is how often the way in which people deal with their illness affects their outcome. In general, patients who 'choose' to accept what is happening to them as much as possible, and who try to carry on as normally as possible, tend to fare better than those patients who worry about and dwell on their illness. Then there are the patients who almost 'set out their own stall' and 'choose' when they will die. The three case studies below describe three very different scenarios.

Lois, in the first case study, chose to accept the fact that she had cancer, and along with this she accepted the changes imposed by the disease, and just got on with her life.

Gully, in the second case study, was slightly different. Diagnosed with a brain tumour, he was very ill following surgery and subsequent treatment, and when he was transferred to the nursing home, it was really felt that he was dying. However, as his treatment began to take effect, he started to improve physically. Mentally, he still thought that he was dying, and his whole attitude was very negative. As described in the case study, he was very reluctant even to get out of bed. So, because he wouldn't help himself, others did it for him. By having case conferences attended by professionals and his family, Gully was gently encouraged to do more. As he found his capabilities improving, he wanted to join in these discussions and to have some say about what happened to him. As he began to realise that he was 'living' rather than 'dying', his attitude began to become more positive, and he started to enjoy his achievements and to build on them.

Pamela, in the third case study, 'chose' her time of departure and amazed everyone by dying exactly as she had predicted.

I have also been amazed by the way that patients with mental disability cope with their illness. Often they do not fully understand what is going on, and so long as they are allowed to remain in a familiar environment, with familiar people around them, these patients often fare really well, even when they have extensive illness and their outlook is expected to be poor. The case studies of Frank and Katy in Chapter 25 are good examples of this type of denial.

CASE STUDY LOIS – THE PATIENT WHO GOT ON WITH LIFE

Lois, an 84-year-old woman, was diagnosed with cancer of the pancreas in November 2006. Unfortunately, her cancer was not operable because of her poor health status, which included heart and thyroid problems. Lois and her family were unsure whether she would live to see Christmas that year, but she did. When I first met Lois, it was 6 months after her diagnosis and she had moved into a care home with nursing staff, as she and her family felt that she was becoming too unwell to cope at home. At the time of my visit, Lois was very comfortable and content. She understood her diagnosis and her poor prognosis, and felt calm and unafraid of approaching death. She did not wish to go back into hospital, but wanted to end her days in the nursing home. She was on a huge amount of medication. This was mainly for her heart and thyroid, but she was also taking morphine for pain. Because of her poor prognosis, I liaised with her GP to have some medications available that could be used via the syringe driver when she deteriorated. I continued to visit Lois periodically over the year, and never failed to be amazed by her cheerfulness and her positive attitude. She was always willing to join in with activities, and liked to keep busy. She was an avid scrabble player, and had formed a group of residents who gathered together to play weekly. When a member of the group became too ill to join in, Lois would try to recruit someone else. She loved sewing and making things, and was busy with a needle whenever I visited. Because of her heart problems, she was on continuous oxygen, but this did not stop her from taking part in fundraising activities for the nursing home, and she was often out on her mobility scooter shaking a tin somewhere to collect money. Every now and then when I visited, she would describe a symptom that was troubling her. However, once I had explained the likelihood of what was causing it and what could be done, she understood and was happy to work with the suggestions made by the doctors and myself. This usually involved increasing her morphine dose and/or adding in another drug. Tiredness was quite a problem for Lois, but although it curbed her energy, she did not let it prevent her from carrying on with her activities. She would choose part of the day to be active, and would then rest for the other part of the day. She had set a goal of finishing a cross-stitch tapestry of a dog as a Christmas present for one of the nurses in the home. However, she was now becoming so tired that after a few stitches she found herself dropping off to sleep. She was prescribed a short course of a steroid called dexamethasone to give her energy and appetite a lift. This helped to give her the boost she needed, and she managed to finish her tapestry, along with many tapestry Christmas cards to be sold on behalf of the home. No one really thought that Lois would survive to a second Christmas, but we all underestimated her determination. As the second Christmas approached, she was determined to go to her family's home for the day. And she did. As I write this case study, it is now nearly 18 months since her diagnosis. As always, no one can predict a person's life expectancy even when they have a life-limiting disease. Overall, however, pancreatic cancer has a poor prognosis, and by the time someone experiences symptoms and undergoes tests, their disease is very often quite advanced. Most people who are diagnosed with pancreatic cancer are told that they may have less than a year to live. Cancer of the pancreas is also often quite uncomfortable, with symptoms such as abdominal pain, sickness and changes in bowel habit. Taking all this on board, Lois is quite an amazing person who, through her own determination and positive action, is living as well as she possibly can alongside her life-limiting illness.

CASE STUDY GULLY – THE PATIENT WHO NEEDED HELP TO START TO LIVE AGAIN

Gully is a 53-year-old man, and is married, with children and grandchildren. He is an avid football supporter, and prior to becoming ill, he enjoyed taking part in outdoor activities such as fishing. I first met him just after Christmas 2005, having been asked to go and see him by the nursing home staff. The nurses told me that Gully had just been discharged to them from hospital, where he had been receiving treatment for a brain tumour. They described his condition as very poorly, and they did not expect him to live for very long. The doctor had visited and told Gully and his family that time was very short. When I saw Gully, he was lying in a darkened room, quite restless and confused, and feeling very nauseated. It was very difficult for him to communicate with me, and even his wife was struggling to understand what he was saying. He looked very poorly and, like the doctor, I did not think that Gully had many days left to live. I advised that a syringe driver should be set up with some medication to relieve his restlessness and nausea. I then went to talk to his wife to explain what was happening, and gently prepared her for the fact that her husband was likely to die within the next few days. However, Gully did not die as expected, and after a few days the syringe driver was discontinued. Although he was still poorly, he was no longer expected to die imminently. Over the next few weeks, Gully continued to improve. He started eating and communicating, and the nurses were trying to encourage him to sit out of bed for a while. It was fairly evident that the loss of movement he had suffered down his right side would not improve much, but he had good movement in his other side, and his senses were intact. His speech continued to improve, and it was becoming easier to understand him. However, despite improving symptomatically, he was becoming quite a challenge for the nurses who were looking after him. He did not want to get out of bed, or to join in any activities. He was eating very well because of the steroids he was taking, and his weight was increasing daily. This was causing a problem with handling and lifting. When he wasn't eating, he would lie in his bed with the sheet pulled up over his head. He even lay covered like this when his family visited. Gully lost faith in the doctor who had told him and his family that he was dying. He linked every ache and pain that he felt directly to his cancer, and most of his conversation with the nurses and myself was about him dying. The nurses and I tried many different ways to engage Gully in activities, but everything we tried was either unsuccessful, or the success was very short-lived because Gully didn't seem to be able to motivate himself enough to do anything that involved 'living.' Although he was on antidepressants, his mood remained low and he was taking many different medications for pain, which he complained about often. He would have liked to go home, but he knew that this was not possible because of his level of dependence and the fact that his wife was still working. However, he was quite settled in the nursing home, and he didn't want to move anywhere else.

I tried to persuade Gully to attend the local day hospice, but although he initially seemed keen, when the time came for him to go, he made excuses as to why he couldn't manage it – such as headaches, or problems with his hearing.

About a year after Gully had been expected to die, the doctor, nurses and I decided that we really had to push for a better quality of life for Gully and his family. I ordered him an electric wheelchair and asked our clinical psychologist, who was newly in post, to see him. We started to have regular multi-disciplinary meetings with Gully's family to discuss his progress, and we called in various other services to help, such as physiotherapists to help to improve his mobility. Once Gully was responding positively, he joined in the meetings and was able to tell us all how he was improving. He started going to the local day hospice – at first just once a week, and then some weeks he started going twice. This time was like a turning point in his life. Within months, Gully was mobilising around the nursing home in his electric wheelchair. The doctor had stopped or reduced a lot of his medication. He came off the steroids completely and started eating sensibly, so his weight decreased. He had both eyes treated for cataracts, and developed an interest in art. He started to draw pictures of all the nurses, and even requested a room change into a room with more natural light.

As I write this case study, it is now two and a half years since I first met Gully, and he continues to keep quite well. He went home to his family for Christmas day, and still attends the day hospice once or twice each week. Gully still has a life-limiting illness, but he is now living with his illness rather than dying from it.

CASE STUDY PAMELA – THE WOMAN WHO PREDICTED WHEN SHE WOULD DIE

Pamela was a 79-year-old woman who was discharged from the local hospice to a nursing home. Although she had cancer in her lung and was quite frail, she was fairly asymptomatic (symptom free) and it was generally expected that she would live for a few weeks. Pamela's eightieth birthday was on Sunday 27 April. Her family planned to celebrate with a party in her room, and Pamela was very much looking forward to this. During the build-up to her party, she became increasingly bright, and the nurses who cared for her shared in her enthusiasm and encouraged her to have her hair done, and to have nail varnish applied to her fingernails. Pamela told the nurses who cared for her that her party was going to be very special, as it was the day before she was going to die. When they asked her what made her think she was going to die the next day, she told them that she was ready to go, but she wanted her family to remember her last day as being happy, and united with everyone she loved. She said that her family would have lovely memories of her last day of life, and that this would help them through their grief. When she was asked whether she had told her family that she was going to die the next day, she said 'Oh yes, but they don't believe me of course.' The day of Pamela's birthday dawned and she was bright and happy. Her family came and went with presents and food, balloons and cards were littered around the room, and every nurse who entered the room was pressed to have a drink or something to eat. Pamela smiled her way through the day, and although she was very tired at the end, she still seemed quite bright – certainly not like someone who was going to die the next day. She kissed all of her visitors and said her goodbyes. She slept peacefully that night and woke as normal the next day to eat her usual breakfast and read her paper. The only difference at that time was that she said she was too tired for her shower, and opted for a bed bath instead. One of the nurses remarked how well she looked and joked that her prediction was wrong. Pamela told her that the day was not yet over. Around 7 pm that evening, Pamela asked for one of her usual painkillers, saying that she had a pain in her 'heart.' The nurse thought that she might have a touch of indigestion, and gave her a drop of antacid medicine as well. Shortly after taking the medicine, Pamela settled down to sleep. At 8.30 pm, when the carer went to check on her, she reported that Pamela looked 'different', and that her breathing sounded strange. One of the trained nurses went to see, and decided that Pamela was dying. She called her family in and as they sat with her, she very peacefully slipped away at 11.50 pm on Monday 28 April.

Remember: When it comes to living and dying, everyone is different. Always be prepared for the unexpected.

REFERENCE

1 Davies E, Higginson IJ, editors. *Palliative Care: the solid facts.* Geneva: WHO Europe; 2004; www.goldstandardsframework.nhs.uk/non-cancer.php (accessed 21/1/2008)

CHAPTER 27

Older people in care homes

Because people are living longer, the incidence of elderly people living with a life-limiting illness is increasing. Older people are often not listened to as individuals, and their experiences of care range from the very good to the very bad. The type of care that they receive is often rather a lottery, and can vary according to their age and where they are living. In addition, for many elderly people, the last months and years of life can involve a lot of ups and downs, with a general overall deterioration that accompanies old age, interspersed with periods of acute illness such as chest infections and urinary tract infections. Communication about their end-of-life care is often limited, leading to less informed choices and less coordination of care. There is often an assumption that deaths in older patients are 'timely' or 'natural', and these people are therefore often not considered to be in need of the special care or support that is given to younger patients. Older people who have diseases other than cancer often suffer from longer periods of dependency and illness, receive less specialist input, and are generally less likely to receive hospice care.

When an elderly person lives in their own home, they generally have more control over their own treatment, taking their medication when and how it feels right for them, using other methods to improve comfort, such as heat pads, hot water bottles, etc., and perhaps indulging in a nip of alcohol throughout the day and/or night. In their own home they can make their own decisions even if, medically, doctors and nurses would not condone what they were doing. However, when an elderly person goes into a care home, much of their independence and choice is lost. Care homes have rules and regulations that must be adhered to in order to satisfy the governing bodies who oversee them. This very often means that an elderly person is not allowed to self-medicate, or to use hot water bottles (in case of scalding), and must rely on a nurse to provide medication, generally when it is the allotted 'medication round' time. In addition, in some care homes, end-of-life care for the elderly may be hampered by inadequate staff training, lack of resources and lack of support for the carers. A colleague of mine, Dr Tim Hunt, has a particular interest in pain in the older person, and has helped out with some of my education sessions on this subject. In an article he wrote on treating pain in the older person, he identified how some carers expressed the view that they are so overwhelmed with work that standards of care are lower than they should be, and consideration of pain becomes of little importance.[1]

Pain and discomfort are felt by the elderly in many ways, but the most commonly experienced pains are usually in joints and limbs, due to arthritis. An older person or a patient with dementia may have long-term memories of childhood pain experiences which were very traumatic or frightening. These memories, which are often tucked away at the back of their mind for many years, can revive in old age, making any current pain or discomfort a frightening experience. However, these types of pain are often not recognised or treated effectively.

Many older people were brought up in a culture that encouraged stoicism – a 'stiff upper lip' – and therefore a lot of elderly patients don't like to complain. This often leads carers to underestimate the discomfort that these patients are experiencing. This situation is worsened by the fact that the elderly often have multiple illnesses, take a number of different medications, and sometimes have difficulty remembering which pill is for which complaint.

Older people differ from the young in the way that they metabolise medication, because their kidney function is less efficient, so they can't clear the medication from their bodies as quickly. In addition, their central nervous system is often more sensitive, which means that some drugs may make them more sleepy or confused. Because of this, they usually need much smaller doses than younger patients.

Older people have a tendency not to take in much fluid during the day, perhaps because they can't reach their drinks, or because they are worried about needing the toilet. This can lead to swallowing problems, or the tablets not being washed down properly, which results in the medication not being absorbed effectively. As a carer, you need to encourage your patient to take plenty of water, preferably while they are sitting upright. Alternatively, it may be better to ask the doctor to prescribe soluble or liquid medication.

Older people are often required to take many different medications (this is described as 'polypharmacy'). What usually happens is that the doctor prescribes medication for a complaint, and then when another complaint is identified, another medication is added without reviewing what that patient is already taking. This process can continue until an elderly person might be taking in excess of 20 different medications daily. Sometimes they do not even know what all the different medications are for. In addition, the elderly are frequently prescribed drugs such as anti-hypertensives to control blood pressure, statins to control cholesterol levels, aspirin to prevent blood clots, and diuretics (water tablets) for fluid retention. There comes a time when a patient no longer needs to be taking all of these medications. Certainly if an elderly patient is entering the end stage of life, they do not need to be taking all of these drugs. As a carer, it is important that you identify this to the doctor so that he can review the patient's current medication, and hopefully stop some or all of the unnecessary drugs.

Given all of the above, care homes are in a unique position to provide care for the elderly who are no longer able to cope in their own home, but it is very important that all of the carers understand the principles of palliative care, along with the differences in the type of care that the elderly require. Carers need to be encouraged to view their very important role in caring for the elderly with pride. To achieve this, it is important that care homes:

➤ raise awareness of the need to recognise the importance of pain in the elderly
➤ ensure that training in palliative care is provided for all levels of care home staff
➤ access communication skills training in how to communicate effectively with residents and their families about death and dying
➤ have access to specialist palliative care staff
➤ have a range of resources to support the provision of palliative care, such as a syringe driver
➤ use one or more supportive care pathways (*see* Chapter 29)
➤ keep clear and comprehensive documentation describing the individual patient's wishes about their future care (advance care planning).

Remember:
➤ Elderly people have a right to be cared for with the same level of care as would be given to younger patients.
➤ Elderly people have many years of life experience behind them that will influence how they are now.
➤ Elderly people may not complain of pain – it is up to you to look, listen and ask.
➤ Elderly people's metabolism is generally slower than that of younger patients, and they should have their medication reviewed regularly to avoid the 'polypharmacy' scenario whereby they end up taking a large number of different medications.

➤ Elderly people often need encouragement to drink more fluid, or need to have their medications changed to a liquid format.

When I am old
Care for me as though I mean the world to you
Talk to me and touch me as if I hear and feel things too
Don't look on my dying as a failure in your care
If you cared and touched and talked to me, I know that you were there
Remember even though I'm old, I still have feelings deep inside
But sometimes when you're old like me they're easier to hide
One day it may be you who is old and needing care
Think where you would like to be and who you would like there.
Though these thoughts are sad to think and may make you want to cry
Put yourself in my shoes. How would you want to die?
When I am old, in need of care, to you this is my plea
Care for me as you would wish your own care to be

Christine Reddall

REFERENCE

1 Hunt T. Treating pain in the older person. *J Pain Palliat Care Pharmacother.* 2006; **20:** 55–7.

CHAPTER 28

Benefits and grants in palliative care

My experience in palliative care has often shown that carers have little or no idea about funding that can be accessed when a person is suffering from a life-limiting illness. Even in a care home, some patients may be eligible to receive a benefit or grant. When a patient is admitted to a care home, a financial assessment will usually have been carried out to determine whether they are eligible for local authority funding. If they are eligible, all available benefits will be accessed and applied for. However, if a patient is paying for their own care, they may not realise what benefits they can receive, and will be reliant upon information given by their carers.

Grants are completely different, and varying sums of money may be granted to a person regardless of where they live if they have a special need.

My experience of benefits and grants is confined to the area of palliative care, so it is important to contact your local benefit agency, or look in the phone book or on the Internet for contact details of charitable organisations, to obtain information about other benefits and grants.

Macmillan grants

A Macmillan grant can only be accessed for patients with a cancer diagnosis. A professional person, such as a Macmillan nurse, district nurse or social worker, can apply for a grant using a special form. These forms should be available from your local Macmillan team. A Macmillan grant is means tested and has to be requested for something specific, such as clothing, special equipment, a holiday, etc. Usually only one grant per year can be awarded, and there is a ceiling on the amount of money that can be granted. The person who is completing the grant application must write a brief scenario explaining why the patient needs the money. Once a grant has been applied for and accepted, it is paid out quite quickly. Unless otherwise requested, it is made payable to the patient by cheque.

Attendance Allowance (A/A) and Disability Living Allowance (DLA)

These are tax-free benefits for people who require care.
➤ Attendance Allowance is a tax-free benefit for people aged 65 years or over who potentially need help with personal care.
➤ Disability Living Allowance is a tax-free benefit for people under 65 years of age who potentially need help with personal care or who have problems with mobility.

Payment is usually made directly to the ill person, but if that person is unable to act for him- or herself, another individual can be appointed to act for them and receive payment. Payment is usually made directly into a bank or building society account.

Payments of these benefits are affected if a person is in an NHS hospital for more than four weeks, or in a care home that is paid for by the state for more than four weeks.

If a person who is applying for either Attendance Allowance or Disability Living Allowance is considered to be 'terminally ill', these benefits can be applied for under the 'special rules.' For the purpose of the benefits agency, 'terminally ill' refers to a person who is suffering from a progressive disease, and whose death can be reasonably expected to occur within six months.

The special rules section of paperwork is included in both Attendance Allowance and Disability Living Allowance packs. If a person is already receiving either of these benefits and *then* they become terminally ill, they can apply by letter to receive the higher payment awarded under the special rules. The special rules paperwork has to be signed by a doctor or by a specialist nurse such as a Macmillan nurse.

Under normal benefit rules, a person has to prove that they need care and also be able to show that they have needed care for a certain length of time before they qualify for either of the above benefits. Under the special rules, there is no such qualifying period and the person does not have to prove how much care they need. This means that much less information is needed on the claim form, and these claims made under the special rules are given priority treatment.

A claim under the special rules can be made either by the person who is ill or by someone acting on their behalf. It is often better if the claim can be completed by someone other than the ill person, as the wording can be quite distressing, especially if that person is not fully aware of the nature of their condition. In this case, it is not necessary for the ill person to sign the form. A doctor or a Macmillan nurse must then complete a special form known as a DS1500. This requires a short medical report about the ill person's condition, which is then sent to the benefits agency along with the claim form.

The Willow Foundation

This is a national charity dedicated to improving the quality of life of seriously ill young adults through the provision of 'special days.' During my visits to care homes, I am aware of many younger patients, especially in homes for the physically and mentally disabled, who would certainly be eligible for a 'special day.'

The Willow Foundation explains that the aim of every special day is to help a young adult, aged 16 to 40 years, who is living with a serious illness to spend quality time with family and/or friends.

Every special day is entirely individual, and is organised in meticulous detail and with the full involvement of the applicant to ensure that it is as enjoyable and stress-free as possible.

The Willow Foundation organises and funds everything involved in the day, including transport, activity fees, tickets and accommodation, where necessary.

Local charities

There are many local charities that may help by providing varying sums of money for people in need. However, because information varies greatly from one area to another, the best approach is to find the contact details of charities in your local phone book or on the Internet.

Contact details for the organisations discussed above can be found in the chapter on 'Further reading, useful websites and other resources' (*see* page 156).

Remember: The information provided in this chapter is intended merely as a guide. Only the information provided on Macmillan grants is applicable to all areas. Other benefits and grants may differ according to the area in which the patient lives.

CASE STUDY   ALAN – MACMILLAN GRANT

Alan was a 54-year-old man with mouth and lung cancer. He had spent much of his life as rather a nomad, going where the fancy took him and often sleeping in the open. Sadly, his diagnosis meant that he had to have a tracheotomy and a feeding tube into his stomach. It was felt that he was too poorly to return to his nomadic life, and he was found a place in a nursing home. Alan knew that his time was limited, and his one wish was to see the sea again before he died. He had no money, and he knew that his illness would prevent him from going to the seaside in the 'normal' way – for example, by car or train. When I told him that it was possible to obtain some money to help him to achieve his wish, he was delighted and said that at last he had something to look forward to. With the help of a Macmillan grant, I was able to organise a private ambulance to take Alan, his friend and a nurse to Bournemouth for the day. There was some money available to spend when he got there, and a hotel was found near to the sea that would provide a room for him to rest in if he needed to do so. Everything was set in place within two weeks, as Alan's condition was deteriorating quite rapidly. Sadly, he died before he managed to make the trip. All of the arrangements were cancelled and the money was returned to Macmillan. However, even though Alan did not make the trip, his anticipation of going to the seaside gave him something to look forward to during his last weeks of life.

CASE STUDY SUE – A SPECIAL DAY

Sue was a 34-year-old woman with learning disability, who had been diagnosed with cancer of the breast. She was a great fan of Cliff Richard, and always talked about going to see him in concert. With help from the Willow Foundation, she was able to attend such a concert with her parents. The foundation organised everything, and even arranged for Sue to meet her idol. For weeks after the event, during the time leading up to her death, Sue talked of little else but the special day on which she met Cliff.

CASE STUDY BEN – A NEW CHAIR

Ben was an elderly man who was living in a care home. He was very frail and had breathing difficulties, which became worse if he lay down, making him feel very breathless and anxious. The carers did everything that they could to try to make him more comfortable at night, such as providing a head rest, extra pillows, etc. Unfortunately, Ben reached the point where he refused to sleep in his bed at night, and would remain in his chair. The carers were concerned because the chair was a very upright one, and they feared for Ben's comfort and safety, as well as the problem of pressure relief. I was asked whether it was possible to obtain a Macmillan grant for some help with buying a recliner chair. However, this was not possible as Ben did not have a cancer diagnosis. I therefore suggested to the carers that they should consider approaching their local charity organisations for help. As a result of doing this, the care home was granted a payment to help them to buy a recliner chair for Ben. This made all the difference to his quality of life, especially at night. He was able to go out with the carers to choose his chair, and when he died some three months later, he left a request that the care home should keep his chair and use it for other residents.

CHAPTER 29

Care pathways in palliative care

There is a huge national drive to encourage all care homes to implement ways of ensuring best practice in providing care for patients with life-limiting illnesses. In the UK, many care homes are using two of the most well-known tools, both of which have been accredited and recognised by the National Institute for Clinical Excellence (NICE). These are the Liverpool Care Pathway (LCP) and the Gold Standards Framework (GSF). There are other tools and pathways that are used in other areas, but as the LCP and the GSF are the most widely used and well known, I am going to focus on them. Where these pathways are implemented in the care homes that I visit, they work extremely well and give the carers confidence and support, as well as ensuring excellent care for the patients.

THE GOLD STANDARDS FRAMEWORK

The Gold Standards Framework, which categorises patients according to their stage of illness, has been around for quite a while in the general community. The patients' care is coordinated by their doctor and other healthcare professionals, such as the district nurse and the Macmillan nurse. The Gold Standards Framework has now been adapted for the care home setting, and this version is known as the Gold Standards Framework for Care Homes (GSFCH). The aim is to ensure that all patients in care homes receive the best palliative care possible as they approach the end of their lives.

The overall aims of the GSFCH programme are as follows:
➤ to improve the quality of care for patients who are nearing the end of their lives
➤ to improve coordination and collaboration with all caring professionals

> to reduce the number of patients who are transferred to hospital in the last stages of life.

The five goals of the GSFCH can be summarised as follows.

> The patient's symptoms are controlled.
> The patient is enabled to choose their preferred place of care in which to spend the last phase of their life.
> The patient feels safe and secure, with fewer crises.
> The carers feel supported, involved, empowered and satisfied.
> There is enhanced confidence and teamwork among the carers, and communication and collaboration with other professionals are maximised.

At the time of writing, approximately 40 care homes across Great Britain have received the Gold Standard Accreditation Award. Four of these homes are in my area of work, and a further two homes in my area are also very close to receiving this award. I feel extremely proud to be associated with them, as the award means that they are homes which provide a recognised, excellent standard of palliative care.

Currently, for a care home to undertake the GSFCH programme, they must register with the central team. Contact details can be found in the chapter on 'Further reading, useful websites and other resources' (*see* page 156). You can also ask your specialist palliative care nurse about the programme.

In order to achieve the Gold Standard Accreditation Award, there is work to be done by the participating care home. There is some additional paperwork involved, and participants are required to attend workshops. However, in my experience, the initial additional work and changes that need to be made are far outweighed by the benefits to everyone involved, especially the patients.

THE LIVERPOOL CARE PATHWAY

The Liverpool Care Pathway is a tool that can be used for all patients who are in their last days of life, irrespective of their primary disease or the cause of their imminent death. The LCP consists of a set of paperwork that replaces all other nursing care documentation and enables measurable outcomes of care. The aim of the pathway is to keep the patient comfortable by controlling their symptoms. It is important to remember that although a patient may be considered to be dying at the time of assessment for the LCP, the situation can change and that patient may 'recover.' This can happen in the elderly in particular, who can become very ill suddenly (for example, during an infection), and then improve, so are no longer imminently dying. If this happens, the patient can be taken off the pathway.

The LCP is implemented by the following criteria.

The multi-professional team must have agreed that the patient is dying, and that two or more of the following criteria apply:

➤ the patient is bed bound
➤ they are semi-comatose
➤ they are only able to take sips of fluids
➤ they are no longer able to take tablets.

These criteria can be altered if the patient under consideration has different needs. For example, some elderly patients may be bed bound and have difficulty taking tablets and fluids, but they may not be imminently dying (*see* case study below).

When a patient is commenced on the LCP, the following are put in place.

➤ Medications are reviewed and all non-essential drugs are discontinued.
➤ Drugs for subcutaneous use are written up according to a set protocol.
➤ All inappropriate medical interventions, such as antibiotics, blood tests and intravenous fluids, are stopped.
➤ All inappropriate nursing interventions, such as washing and 2-hourly turning, are stopped.
➤ If it is needed, a syringe driver is set up within 4 hours of a doctor's order.
➤ The care plan is explained to and understood by the patient if possible, as well as the family and/or friends.
➤ Religious and/or spiritual needs are assessed with the patient and family.
➤ It is documented how the family or other contacts want to be informed of the patient's impending or actual death.
➤ The patient's family and/or friends are given information about facilities such as accommodation, car parking, access to refreshments, etc.

After death:

➤ the general practitioner is notified of the patient's death
➤ the patient is laid out according to protocol
➤ the family or another person who was close to the patient is given information on what happens after the death – for example, registering the death, collecting the patient's property, etc.
➤ any other advice and information, such as a bereavement leaflet, is offered to each of the bereaved individuals.

As you are reading this, some of you will no doubt be thinking 'Well, we do all that when someone is dying.' What the LCP does is to ensure that 'all the boxes are ticked', and because of this, everyone should be providing the same standard of care and nothing should be missed.

There are two ways of implementing the LCP. The formal way is by registering with the central team, as is done for the GSF. Again, there is additional work to do and paperwork to complete. Alternatively, the LCP can be implemented informally by downloading the paperwork from the LCP website. However, you may need someone experienced in the LCP to go through the paperwork with you, until you become familiar with it. LCP contact details are given in the chapter on 'Further reading, useful websites and other resources' (*see* page 156).

CASE STUDY SUSAN – USING A CARE PATHWAY

(The following case study was kindly supplied by one of the care homes for which I provide input. This care home provided excellent support for Susan and her family, and I was not involved in her care.)

Susan was a 79-year-old woman who was admitted to hospital following a severe stroke. Because she had major difficulties with swallowing, the decision was taken to insert a feeding tube into her stomach. Susan was unable to be cared for in her own home, and was transferred to a care home with nursing staff. The use of the Gold Standards Framework and the Liverpool Care Pathway was well established in that home. The nurse who admitted her explained the GSF programme to Susan and her family, but felt that there was no need to mention the LCP at this stage. Susan's family were given a letter to take away that explained how the GSF would help with her care. Each week, Susan's key carer would discuss any changes with Susan's doctor, and these would be implemented quickly. Susan was completely dependent on two carers for all of her needs, and because she was more comfortable in bed, this is where she was nursed, using pressure-relieving aids and handling equipment. For the first month, Susan was quite stable and comfortable, but she then started to deteriorate. It was noted that she was becoming more sleepy and that she seemed to be less willing to be 'bothered' with her care. Within a few days she developed a chest infection. Susan had completed an advance care plan that had been signed by her doctor, and her wish was that she should not be given any treatment if it was felt that she was entering the end stage of her life. The opinion of all of the professionals involved was that Susan was dying, and that the sole aim of her care should now be to ensure her comfort. Her family were in full agreement with this decision. The team of carers agreed that Susan was dying, and decided that it was time to use the Liverpool Care Pathway. However, the set criteria for using the LCP did not 'fit' in Susan's case. She had been bed bound since her admission, and because she was fed by tube, the criteria 'only able to take sips of fluids' and 'no longer able to take tablets' did not apply to her. Because she was increasingly sleepy, 'semi-comatose' was the only criterion that applied. However, because the care home staff were very experienced with the LCP, they set and agreed their own criteria as follows:

- Susan was semi-comatose.
- Without the feeding tube she would be unable to take tablets and fluids.
- She had a chest infection that she did not want to have treated, and which was likely to get worse.

After these criteria had been agreed, Susan's family were informed and involved in the process. Susan was too poorly to be involved in decision making, but had already made her wishes and funeral plans known. In accordance with the process, all unnecessary medication was stopped. However, because of the feeding tube, necessary liquid medicines could still be administered via this route, so there was no need to change the route of her painkillers to subcutaneous administration. The only subcutaneous medication prescribed in anticipation was hyoscine, to control secretions. All unnecessary medical and nursing interventions were stopped and Susan was checked regularly, according to the LCP paperwork, for any symptoms such as pain, agitation, respiratory tract secretions, nausea or vomiting. She was given regular mouth care, and the family also helped with this. The family stated that they wanted to be contacted at any time of the day or night if there was any change in Susan's condition, but in fact a family member was always present. Two days after commencing the LCP, the carers noticed that Susan's condition was changing. Her breathing was becoming laboured and her skin was tinged blue. They suggested to the family member present that Susan seemed to be entering the final few hours of her life. The rest of the family were alerted, and Susan died very peacefully soon afterwards with all her family around her. Susan's after death care was carried out in accordance with the LCP 'after death' guidelines. Her family were given the necessary information and helped to sort out what they needed to do. They were given a leaflet offering information on bereavement support and offered a telephone call from the care home in a few days to see how they were coping.

CHAPTER 30

Advance care planning

There is currently much talk about advance care planning, and it is increasingly being promoted and discussed in the UK, reflecting changes in recent legislation, such as the Mental Capacity Act.[1] It is anticipated that it will be an important key part of the new NHS End of Life Care Strategy.[2]

When a patient is receiving palliative care, it is helpful and reassuring to all concerned, not least the patient, to know what their preferences and wishes are in relation to their future care. In this chapter I shall briefly describe what is meant by advance care planning, and will then direct you to where you can find more information on this in the chapter on 'Further reading, useful websites and other resources' (*see* page 156).

The following information has been extracted and adapted from the Gold Standards Framework website section on advance care planning.[3]

Advance care planning (ACP) is the term used to describe the process of discussing and planning ahead – for example, in anticipation of some deterioration in a patient's condition. It involves discussion and documentation of the patient's wishes. Family members and/or friends can be involved if the patient wants them to be. The type of wishes and preferences that might be discussed may include the following:

➤ where the patient wants to be cared for at the end of their life
➤ how they would prefer to be cared for – for example, fears expressed about dying alone
➤ the type of treatment and care that they want, or do not want
➤ funeral arrangements.

There are two specific areas within advance care planning.
1 **Advance Statement/Statement of Wishes.** This involves discussion of the patient's preferences, wishes and likely plans for their future. It is not legally

147

binding, but is invaluable in determining planned provision of care.
2 **Advance Decision.** This clarifies refusal of treatment or what patients do *not* wish to happen. It involves assessment of mental competency to make that decision at the time and, when accurately formulated, it can be legally binding. It also strengthens the role of the Lasting Power of Attorney to enable a nominated proxy person to make decisions about the patient's medical as well as social welfare.

Once an advance care plan has been drawn up, it is important that it is reviewed regularly, as a person's wishes and preferences may change.

Do Not Attempt Resuscitation (DNAR) orders are always a very contentious issue in care homes, and one that I am frequently asked about.

Policies and paperwork for DNAR orders differ from one area to another, and your local NHS trust should have a policy on DNAR decisions, as well as guidance on how these are recorded. Some areas also have a DNAR template for the recording of these decisions.

Many care homes already do advance care planning, but it is my experience that many carers feel uncomfortable asking patients sensitive questions about their future care and funeral arrangements. However, many elderly people actually welcome such a discussion and feel grateful that the carer can discuss these important issues with them. You may find some of the following phrases helpful when opening up such a conversation:

> 'It would be helpful to us to know a little more about the sort of things you would like or not like to happen while you are with us.'

> 'How do you see your future now that you are with us?'

> 'If the time comes when you need more care, where would you like to be looked after?'

> 'What do you think your family would prefer?'

> 'It's sometimes comforting to know that your affairs are sorted out. Do you need any help with organising this?'

For the patient who has communication difficulties (for example, due to dementia), or who is too ill to communicate, the process of ascertaining their wishes becomes a challenge. Here it is important for you to be aware of the correct policy and procedure for dealing with such a situation. Most of you will no doubt be familiar with the recently revised Mental Capacity Act, and your manager should be the person to consult about this.

Remember: Talking about patients' wishes with regard to their care in the future is not easy. However, if we want to help them to receive the best care possible according to their wishes, it is vital that we as carers listen to what our patients want, and take time to plan and record this as early in their care as possible. This helps to ensure that there is more pro-active planning, which should in turn lead to fewer crises, enabling the patient to be cared for according to their wishes, and in their place of choice.

REFERENCES

1 Nuffield Foundation. *Advance Care Planning in Care Homes. Final Report.* London: Nuffield Foundation; 2008.
2 www.goldstandardsframework.nhs.uk/advanced.care.php (accessed 1/2/2008)
3 www.goldstandardsframework.nhs.uk/advanced.care.php (accessed 1/2/2008)

CHAPTER 31

Palliative care education

Currently, palliative care training in care homes is encouraged, but it is not mandatory. Before I became a Macmillan nurse for care homes, the care homes in my area received very little in the way of palliative care education. They seldom heard about external education sessions, such as those held at the hospice, and those carers who had a special interest in palliative care often had to find and fund a suitable course or distant learning programme themselves. Since I have been in this role, care homes have requested many training sessions and I have been happy to help them out with whatever area of palliative care they want to learn about. I have found that it is easier to do the training in house, as it is often difficult for carers to get time out to attend training courses. I have also found a tremendous willingness and enthusiasm among the carers when engaged in training sessions, and they often comment that learning about palliative care increases their confidence when giving care at the end of life. I send twice-yearly newsletters to each care home in the area, in which I inform them of the courses and study days that are available. I also include them in a mailing list about education that is available locally. I am often asked to provide training on subjects such as the following:

➤ My role as Macmillan nurse for care homes.
➤ Death and dying.
➤ What is palliative care?
➤ Syringe driver training.
➤ Answering difficult questions.
➤ Pain management for untrained staff.
➤ Management of the patient's last days of life.
➤ Management of nausea and vomiting.
➤ What is cancer?
➤ Management of constipation.

➤ Management of breathlessness.
➤ The Gold Standards Framework (GSF).
➤ Drugs in palliative care.

If the care home is caring for a patient with a specific diagnosis, such as a certain type of cancer, I encourage them to invite me to visit so that we can talk about that patient and discuss the possible signs and symptoms they might observe.

During the time that I have been in post, care homes have been increasingly caring for patients with complex palliative care needs, using syringe drivers and generally being expected to provide much more nursing care. In order to look after these patients, carers need to receive palliative care training. If as a carer you are reading this and are unsure how to access training, a good place to start would be your local hospice or Macmillan team. I have included details of some relevant courses that are available nationally in the chapter on 'Further reading, useful websites and other resources' (*see* page 157).

CHAPTER 32

Looking after yourself

Providing palliative care for patients in the final stage of their lives can be very draining, especially when we know that the patient is not going to recover. When working in a care home, staff resources are often less than ideal, and most days tend to be rushed, due to the need to fit everything in and provide care for patients ranging from those who are quite well to those who are dying. Also, because many people live in care homes for weeks, months or even years, they do become part of the care home 'family', and when they become poorly and eventually die, it is not unusual for the carers to experience a sense of loss. We are only human, and it is very easy to become more 'attached' to some patients than others, and the death of these patients undoubtedly leaves us with an emotional scar. Unfortunately, in a care home there often isn't time to grieve, as there is always someone else who needs to be cared for, and a vacant bed is usually quickly filled by another patient.

Some of the possible reasons why carers struggle physically and emotionally may be related to the following:

➤ lack of training and support
➤ carers being unaware of the potential benefits of existing services, such as the Macmillan nurse, or the counselling service
➤ poor communication, either within the team or between the various services provided
➤ exploration of feelings may take too much time
➤ unrealistic expectations – carers expect their involvement to have a positive effect on the health and happiness of the patient. However, this may be unrealistic for patients who are suffering from a life-limiting disease
➤ personal survival – it is often easier to try to forget by carrying on with physical jobs, rather than talking and thinking about the patient who has died.

So how can you help yourself?

➤ Education and training. It is often all too easy to opt for more 'defined' training, such as symptom control issues. However, don't underestimate the importance of any training or support that helps you to look after yourself. After all, if you don't look after yourself, it will be difficult for you to look after others.

➤ Know your limits – you can only do so much in a day. You should also respect the knowledge that you have, and if you don't feel you are the right person to deal with an issue, find someone who is.

➤ Recognise your limitations in providing care for others when you are under particular stress.

➤ Don't be afraid to ask for support.

➤ Take time out. This is not always easy when you are busy, but try!

➤ Be flexible and give each other 'permission' to take care of yourselves – for example, if you notice that a colleague is struggling, send her off for a cup of tea.

➤ Try to switch off at the end of the day. I used to find this very hard to do, and often drove home with my head buzzing. I eventually learned to identify a 'landmark' not too far from my place of work (usually an island), and when I reached this, I would make a conscious effort to take in a deep breath, open the window if the weather permitted, and turn on the radio. This took some practice initially, but I am very good at it now!

➤ Reflective practice – this is an extremely useful exercise, especially after a patient has died, or after a difficult period of caring. It basically involves getting the team of carers together and talking through the situation. It can be done informally, but it is very helpful to ask a professional, such as a Macmillan nurse, to come in and help you with this. The important thing is to pick out the positive aspects as well as the negative ones. No matter how awful a situation may have been, there is nearly always something good to focus on.

Remember: It can be difficult to notice your own burnout until you become ill. You are only human, and therefore you are likely to experience a wide range of emotions. Accept these feelings for what they are and for what they feel like. Experiencing negative feelings such as frustration or anger about your responsibilities, or the people with whom you are working, is normal. It does not mean that you are a bad person or a bad caregiver. Feeling sad when someone has died is also normal, regardless of whether you were caring for them professionally or personally.

Further reading, useful websites and other resources

What is palliative care?

➤ Penson J and Fisher R (eds). *Palliative Care for People with Cancer.* London: Edward Arnold; 1991.

➤ Hockley J and Clarke D (eds). *Palliative Care for Older People in Care Homes.* Buckingham: Open University Press; 2002.

➤ Addington-Hall JM and Higginson IJ (eds). *Palliative Care for Non-Cancer Patients.* New York: Oxford University Press; 2001.

➤ Fallon M and Hanks G (eds). *ABC of Palliative Care.* 2nd edn. Oxford: Blackwell; 2006.

➤ Worthington R. *Ethics in Palliative Care.* Oxford: Radcliffe Publishing; 2005.

What is a hospice?

➤ www.nhpco.org

➤ Ward D (ed.). *Hospice and Palliative Care Directory.* London: Hospice Information; 2006.

What is cancer?

➤ www.cancerbackup.org.uk

➤ www.cancerresearch.uk.org

What is a syringe driver?

➤ Dickman A, Schneider J and Varga J. *The Syringe Driver, Continuous subcutaneous infusions in palliative care.* 2nd edn. Oxford: Oxford University Press; 2005.

➤ Twycross R, Wilcock A and Thorp S. *PCF1: Palliative Care Formulary.* Oxford: Radcliffe Medical Press; 1999.

➤ Kaye P. *A-Z Pocket Book of Symptom Control.* 2nd edn. Northampton: EPL Publications; 2003.

Symptom control

➤ Twycross R. *Symptom Management in Advanced Cancer.* 2nd edn. Oxford: Radcliffe Medical Press; 1997.
➤ Saunders C and Sykes N (eds). *The Management of Terminal Malignant Disease.* 3rd edn. London: Edward Arnold; 1993.
➤ Kaye P. *A-Z Pocket Book of Symptom Control.* 2nd edn. Northampton: EPL Publications; 2003

Difficult questions

➤ Lugton J. *Communicating with Dying People and Their Relatives.* Oxford: Radcliffe Medical Press; 2002.
➤ Buckman R. *I Don't Know What to Say.* London: Macmillan London Limited and Papermac; 1998.
➤ Kaye P. *Breaking Bad News: a ten step approach.* Northampton: EPL Publications; 1995.

The dying process

➤ Ellershaw J and Wilkinson S (eds). *Care of the Dying: a pathway to excellence.* Oxford: Oxford University Press; 2003.

After death

➤ Farrell M. *The Facts of Death: coping when someone dies.* St Edmundsbury Press; 1991.

Dementia

➤ Dementia Helpline, Alzheimer Scotland. Tel: 0800 808 3000.
➤ MacKinlay M. *Working with Dementia: a pocket book for care staff.* Funded by Millennium Awards 2004. Single copies free to care staff from Dementia Helpline, Tel: 0808 808 3000.
➤ www.alzscot.org
➤ Murphy J and Cameron L. *Talking Mats: a resource to enhance communication.* Stirling: AAC Research Team. Tel: 01786 467645.

Learning disability

➤ www.mencap.org.uk
➤ www.bild.org.uk
➤ The Disdat tool is a distress assessment tool designed by St Oswald's

Hospice to help health professionals to identify distress cues in people who, due to cognitive impairment or physical illness, have severely limited communication skills. It can be downloaded from www.mencap.com/document.asp?id=1476

Older people in care homes

➤ Hockley J and Clarke D (eds). *Palliative Care for Older People in Care Homes.* Buckingham: Open University Press; 2002.
➤ Lilley R, Lambden P and Gillies A. *Medicines Management for Residential and Nursing Homes.* Oxford: Radcliffe Publishing; 2007.
➤ *Nursing and Residential Care.* Monthly journal for care assistants, nurses and managers. MA Healthcare Ltd, St Jude's Church, Dulwich Road, London SE24 0PB. Tel: 020 7738 5454.

Benefits and grants

➤ Macmillan grants. Telephone helpline: 0808 801 0304.
www.macmillan.org.uk/get.support/financial_help/financial_help.aspx
➤ Benefits. Telephone helpline: 0800 882200.
www.patient.co.uk/showdoc/23069010/
➤ Willow Foundation Special Days for the 16s to 40s: Willow Foundation, Willow House, 18 Salisbury Square, Hatfield, Herts AL9 5BE. Tel: 01707 259777. Website: www.willowfoundation.org.uk/home.shtml
Email: info@willowfoundation.org.uk

Care pathways

➤ Gold Standards Framework (GSF) Central Team, c/o Walsall PCT, North Walsall, Park View Centre Brownhills, Chester Road, Walsall WS8 7JB. Website: www.goldstandardsframework.nhs.uk/care-homes.php
Email: info@goldstandardsframework.co.uk
Telephone helpline: 01922 604666.
➤ Liverpool Care Pathway (LCP) Central Team UK, c/o Directorate of Specialist Palliative Care, First Floor, Linda McCartney Centre, Royal Liverpool University Hospital, Prescot Street, Liverpool L7 8XP. Tel: 0151 706 2273/2274.
Website: www.mcpcl.org.uk/liverpool-care-pathway
Email: lcp.enquiries@rlbuht.nhs.uk

Advance care planning

➤ www.endoflifecareforadults.nhs.uk/eolc/acp.htm
➤ Resuscitation Council UK; www.resus.org.uk/pages/dnar.htm

Palliative care education

➤ Website for care homes; www.pcchnetwork.org.uk
➤ Regnard C (ed.). *Helping the Patient with Advanced Disease: a workbook.* Oxford: Radcliffe Medical Press; 2004.
➤ Palliative care course – VRQ level
  Website: www.strawberryrecruitment.co.uk.com/clients-1m.php
  Tel: 0845 094 3110.
➤ Foundations in Palliative Care: a programme of facilitated learning for care home staff. Macmillan Cancer Relief. Available from Macmillan Resources Line on 01344 350310 or via www.professionalresources.org. uk/Macmillan

Initiatives to enhance patient care and carer support in care homes

During my work as a Macmillan nurse for care homes, some of the initiatives that I have found worked well in care homes in my area are listed below, with a brief description of each. All of these ideas were worked on alongside some of my highly regarded Macmillan colleagues, and supported by carers from the care homes.

Palliative care resource booklet for care homes

I compiled two booklets, one for palliative care in general care homes and the other for care homes for people with learning disabilities. Each booklet is about 40 pages in length and includes my contact details, information about palliative care, symptoms in palliative care and the last days of life. The booklets are spiral bound, but with hindsight should have been loose leaf, as some of the information has since changed.

Setting up a care home website

I am aware that there are many excellent initiatives around to enhance the care given in care homes. Unfortunately, due to the very way that care homes work, it is not always easy for them to share ideas.

I used some of the money I received for education in care homes to set up a care home network, supported and helped by a colleague who also assisted with the finances. This network can be accessed via www.pcchnetwork.org. uk. The aim of the network is for palliative care professionals like me to share ideas and projects that help to enhance the palliative care that is provided in care homes. The members of the network meet twice yearly, and the content of each meeting is posted on the website. Carers who work in care homes have their own section on this website, and once they have signed up they can interact with others. Questions and answers can be posted here. Sadly, there are still many care homes that do not yet have Internet access.

Newsletters

Twice yearly, I compile and send out a newsletter to every care home in my area. This includes such items as the latest news, changes in contact details, education sessions, awards, good practice, etc.

Syringe drivers

Many care homes that have nursing staff now use syringe drivers quite often. However, not all of the homes have ready access to one when it is needed. I encouraged a number of homes to purchase their own syringe driver, and by 'buying in bulk' I was able to negotiate a considerable discount from the manufacturer. With regard to the regular training necessary to ensure safe use of the syringe driver, I worked with a colleague and the local university on developing a DVD/video teaching aid. This incorporates the description and working of the three syringe driver/pumps described in this book, and also discusses the drugs that can be used. For more information on this teaching aid, please contact the author of this book.

Each care home that owns and uses a syringe driver is encouraged to keep a syringe driver resource box with the following contents (some of the documents are local to my area):

Syringe driver

Check service date.

- Instruction manual for syringe driver/pump.
- Plastic cover or appropriate lock box.
- A selection of infusion lines.
- Two 9V batteries.
- A selection of 10-ml, 20-ml and 30-ml luer lock syringes.
- Needles.
- Red rate setting key.
- Paper clips in case key is lost.
- Labels.
- Clear adhesive dressings.
- Warwickshire Community Pharmacy Palliative Care Service document (local document).
- West Midland Guidelines (local document).
- Prescription chart.
- Syringe driver checklist.

➤ Drug compatibilities.
➤ Pathways for prescribing and administration.
➤ Symptom control algorithms.
➤ Servicing guidelines.
➤ Palliative care service contact details.

Index